The
Path
to
Cure

The Whole Art of Healing

Allyson McQuinn, HD(RHom)

Book Coach Press

The Path to Cure: The Whole Art of Healing

By Allyson McQuinn

Copyright © 2004, Allyson McQuinn

Published by Book Coach Press
Ottawa, Ontario, Canada
www.BookCoachPress.com

Allyson McQuinn
Arcanum Wholistic Clinic
www.arcanum.ca
amcquinn@arcanum.ca

National Library of Canada Cataloguing in Publication

McQuinn, Allyson, 1963-
    The path to cure : the whole art of healing / Allyson McQuinn.

Includes bibliographical references.
ISBN 0-9735207-0-1

1. McQuinn, Allyson, 1963- 2. Homeopathy. I. Title.

RX76.M38 2004   615.5'32   C2004-902091-9

For Jordan,
your strength and courage
led me to the dark side of the moon
and beyond

The truth about our childhood is stored up in our body,

and although we can repress it, we can never alter it.

Our intellect can be deceived, our feelings manipulated,

our perceptions confused,

and our body tricked with medication.

But some day the body will present its bill,

for it is as incorruptible as a child

who, still whole in spirit,

will accept no compromises or excuses,

and it will not stop tormenting us

until we stop evading the truth.

Alice Miller

Table of Contents

Foreword

The greatest story ever told is the story of the journey of each of us to find ourselves. This journey is often an arduous one, requiring one to travel into the darkest reaches of the soul and spirit, a journey that Joseph Conrad termed going "into the heart of darkness" and Scripture calls "the valley of the shadow of death." For that reason, it is a journey seldom taken, the "narrow path" to the Kingdom of God.

The story of mankind is not so much the evolution of matter as modern, material science would have us believe, but the evolution of human consciousness, for matter is but the stage against which the struggle between the forces of light and dark are thrown up, like a Javanese shadow puppet play. Life, as Goethe, the great 17th century scientist and poet, contemporary of the founder of homeopathy and Heilkunst, stated, is but the result of the "deeds and sufferings" of these polar forces. We are born into this world not simply as a random fact, but as a soul-spiritual being with a particular mission to evolve further in our consciousness and spiritual purpose. Health then becomes not so much a matter of removing symptoms at the physical level, a kind of negative state of no pain, as a positive state of greater inner awareness and dedication to the expression of one's deepest desires and fulfillment. This is what Heilkunst is all about.

A true system of medicine must be grounded in natural law and must also remove the true causes of disease, which lie often at the level or our energetic existence, up into our soul and spiritual dimension. It is not enough to remove symptoms if this removal is a result of suppression. Our symptoms are a language of the body mirroring the state of our soul-spiritual being. We can shoot the messenger so to speak, but then we lose the gift hidden in the dark recesses of our pain. If we remove our pain by removing the deeper cause according to natural law, we find that we receive the gift of a deeper awareness and realization about ourselves and our purpose here on earth. We become more alive in terms of our senses and our spiritual capacity.

Heilkunst is a German term for the "art of rendering one whole" or, in its more esoteric sense, the "art and science of salvation." It is not a religious conversion, but a profound scientific system that emerged out of the Romantic Movement in Western evolution of using natural law to convert disease and imbalance in our being into light forces so that we can unfold the divine potential that exists within each of us. It was founded by Dr. Samuel Hahnemann, a man of genius like Goethe. Dr. Hahnemann's name is more readily associated with homeopathic medicine. Homeopathy is but one aspect of this remarkable system of rational medicine termed Heilkunst, which encompasses diet, nutrition, energy and manipulation therapies, essences, psychotherapy, medicine proper and also the transforming of belief into knowledge.

Allyson's story is remarkable precisely as all stories of those treated by Heilkunst are, because she had the courage to undertake the long journey of the soul to find herself. While it is a difficult journey it is also one of liberation and self-worth, of transforming the traumas and weight of the past into the joy and light of the present. It is a story that we all contain within us to varying degrees if we are willing to undergo it. While we may at first be seeking only to remove the pain, we soon learn that it involves as much the discovery of what we have lost. In the process, the pain leaves and a deep inner peace and contentment emerges; one that allows us to face the challenges of life with hope, trust and love, instead of dread, suspicion and fear. Allyson has gone further in her journey, as her self-discovery has led her to study Heilkunst at the Hahnemann College for Heilkunst in Ottawa, Canada so that she might share what she has achieved and learned with others who wish to undertake the same journey of self-discovery.

I thank her for being willing to share the details of her journey with others in this book. It is never easy to let others into the private recesses of our soul. I also thank her for having devoted her energy and thoughts to becoming a Doctor of Medical Heilkunst. It takes courage and a profound level of inner health to step out and to daily confront disease and suffering in others. The world and those who come into contact with her during her life will be the better for it.

Rudi Verspoor, FHCH, HD(RHom) DMH
Dean, Hahnemann College for Heilkunst
Director, Hahnemann Center for Heilkunst
Trustee, Hahnemann Center for Heilkunst Trust

Acknowledgements

I would like to acknowledge the individuals who have contributed to the creation of this book. Rudolf Verspoor for enlivening Dr. Samuel Hahnemann's system of homeopathic medicine therapeutically and for giving a clear succinct voice to Steven Decker's research. Rudi denies any genius on his part, but there is good reason why Patty tapes his murmurings in sleep and we all hang on "the logos" rendered from his lips. Not everyone can take a 200-year-old sleeping giant, contain it in principles, and waltz with it dynamically around the room. Through living examples, students actually envision leading the next dance. Rudi's truth, love and support during my own treatment helped put my derailed train back on track. Truly a 20th century Heilkunst Sherpa guide with a sound map.

Admittedly, Steven Decker's scope and imagination is largely beyond what I can assimilate in my lifetime. I have imagined him many times having enlivened conversations with Dr. Hahnemann, Goethe and Rudolf Steiner. By peering through the portal provided by his organizing lens, we can feel our breath momentarily taken from us. The infinite wisdom of Nature and those Romantics who could perceive her depths keep us enthralled and hungering for more. Poets and scientists residing in the same resonant world speaking in German sentences longer than the distance between Ottawa and California!

Patty Smith was the first loving beacon extended to Jordan and myself when I felt beyond forsaken. Her endless source of knowledge and honesty guided my beleaguered mind and body towards the borderland of health and well-being. Her guiding hand was always one step ahead of my soul.

A special thanks to Linda Lou (Mom) McQuinn, Rick Glatt, Linda Clifford, Catherine Shields, Ansley Simpson, Serena Williamson Andrew at Book Coach Press, Donald Lanouette and Venetia Diamond for their editing, wisdom and guidance.

A very heartfelt thank you to Jeff Korentayer as I have grown monumentally in the time we've rediscovered each other. I look forward to further exploration of infinite resources through resonance.

My love and appreciation to Jordan and Adie who expect nothing less than "The Path to Cure" from their mother who rightfully demand my health and well-being. If we listen to the butterflies flying in formation in our children … it is all they are asking of us.

Allyson McQuinn

CHAPTER 1

JORDAN'S BIRTH

My son, Jordan, was born seven weeks prematurely. After my water broke at 32 weeks, I held onto him for another week as his watery home leaked down my legs. From the numerous ultrasounds, we could see that he was generating a pocket of amniotic fluid around his mouth and he was effectively breathing it in and out of his lungs. His heartbeat and movements were closely monitored 24 hours a day. As I lay in bed listening for his little voice to tell me what was to come next, I tapped out his heartbeat on the hard-covered books I was reading. I was waiting for the rhythm of our one parallel life to divide into two.

The doctors, after telling me that my baby would weigh around four and a half pounds at birth, administered steroid shots into my hip to encourage his lung development. Their main concerns were his size and ability to breathe effectively on his own. The pediatrician, specializing in premature births, said that the chances were excellent that my baby would be a "fully operational model" and the last four weeks in utero were solely about weight gain and putting the finishing touches on lung development. I turned over on the rubber mattress, listened to my baby's heartbeat and waited.

On the fourth day in hospital, my husband wheeled me down to the special care nursery so that we could meet a baby of similar weight and development to ours. This is a foreign world known by only a few. The nursing staff walked around calmly, monitoring alarms that blared when a baby forgot to breathe. I was shocked beyond belief to see a baby that was just over one pound. He looked more like an organism from another planet than someone's child. He was hooked up to enough monitoring equipment that I'm sure the wires alone weighed ten times what he did.

I saw healthy quadruplets lying in open incubators all in a row, waiting to go home the next day. I saw a ten-pound infant which I thought looked like an oversized baby piglet; big, round and very pink. He was being treated for having swallowed too much muconium on his way out into the world.

This was the sequestered ward for little ones with birth defects, and my baby was going to be numbered among them. I spotted a small sleeping baby in an enclosed incubator at the far side of the room. Hooked up to a variety of equipment, she weighed four pounds six ounces and had been born the day before. I'll never forget the sensation creep up my spine as I realized that there was nothing normal about giving birth to such a tiny form.

The life principle did not appear to be fully animated in these petite beings. It was if they had been plucked too soon, their one natural energetic chord of life-support severed and replaced by a multitude of plastic tubes and metal wires. These babies appeared exposed, vulnerable and clearly out of their domain. I could see in the eyes of their mothers an acknowledgment of their present reality, a gaping chasm that separated them from their expectations of childbirth.

Jordan emerged into the world three days later by cesarean section after his heart rate went up to 200 beats per minute. His Apgar scores weren't on any chart as he was ripped from my body. He was small, blue and not breathing. He was rushed like a little football to another room. The rhythm of the pounding heartbeat finally broken, I began to wait for news. As I was being sewn up, someone mentioned that he was a boy. My Jordan was now on his own, defining his own terms.

Allyson McQuinn

When Jordan was brought to me wrapped in a blanket, I held his tiny little body in my two hands and greeted the old-looking face that stared back at me. He appeared peaceful, like a baby rabbit that had been rescued after some malevolent force had entered his warren. I held his very still body next to mine and felt his warmth. This was my baby, but I wasn't sure what to do with him. The nurse rescued me. He was expected in the Special Care Nursery for tests and monitoring. I reluctantly let go of my little bunny and waited for further instructions. As my exhausted husband curled up in the bed next to mine, we stared blankly at each other. Where would this road lead us?

A few days later, free of the tube collecting my urine, I arduously made my way to the bathroom on my own. A self-administered morphine pump had become my constant pain-relieving companion. I learned to pump the colostrum from my breasts every two hours, day and night, and to maneuver my wheelchair slowly down the long corridor to feed my baby. I held him next to my awaiting nipple and simultaneously pushed the syringe full of drug-permeated milk down into his nose tube.

Miraculously, by the fifth day all of Jordan's tubes were gone. We weren't out of the woods though, for soon he needed bilirubin lights on his very jaundiced skin.

After four days, I developed an infection in my wound and they had to reopen me. When the freezing around the wound wouldn't take, my agonized screams were augmented by my need to release some of the pent up emotional anguish I had held steadfastly within over the past couple of weeks. The intern packed me with gauze and started an intravenous drip with nine different antibiotics. I felt nauseous and dizzy, and sweated profusely 24 hours a day. The nurses changed my sheets three times each night. My husband slept upright in a chair by my side as I slipped in and out of delirium. By the second week, I still had not passed stool, so I stood in a line in the hall each morning to receive my ineffectual stool softener as I was effectively holding on to everything. Little did I realize how much this was a harbinger of things to come, not so much for me, but for my precious son.

I was so numb, so bewildered, so emotionally shut down that I didn't think about what all these substances were doing to me, let alone to my premature baby who lay waiting for the next syringe full of my medicine-contaminated milk. In addition, I had been on antibiotics twice during pregnancy as a last ditch effort to combat sinus infections so severe that I wanted to bang my head against a wall to relieve the pressure.

I was finally released from hospital and went home without my son. I set alarms around the clock to mechanically pump my breasts in order to encourage my milk to come in. In between the two visits a day from a home care nurse who was still attending to my open wound, I would rush to the hospital with my little bottles of two to three ounces of butter-like colostrum and feed my baby who was just starting to suckle effectively. It was one of the most dismal and pitiable times in my life. I felt so torn between caring for myself so I could heal, and mothering him. I ached that I was not with him always. I wondered if he would suffer issues of abandonment as a result of the circumstances. This increased my anxiety tenfold.

CHAPTER 2

COLIC AND CONSTIPATION

I finally brought Jordan home on a glorious August morning, three arduous weeks after he'd been born. I couldn't believe that he was all mine and I didn't have to share him with a whole team of nurses. I started to heal much more quickly and he began to nurse enough to bring my milk in. He was gaining an average of a pound and a half a week. We scheduled his Brit Milah four weeks after he arrived home. This is the ritual circumcision which represents the first covenant observed by Jews. Although I was not born Jewish, I had studied for three years and converted to Judaism just prior to marrying my husband. I had also agreed to raise our children in the Jewish faith.

Within two weeks, while Jordan continued to grow, something new emerged. Colic! Jordan's case was particularly severe; he cried constantly, day and night. He fed every hour and a half to two hours and we walked the floor until the carpet was worn. My husband would often go to work and leave both Jordan and I sobbing in the rocking chair. Nurses from the post-natal class came to my home to see how I was making out as I had spent the classes pacing the hall outside as Jordan wailed non-stop, raging against an unseen enemy.

I resorted to gripe water and ignored the alcohol content. We walked around the neighbourhood for hours with him in a stroller. He was so overwhelmed by the "outside" that he would close his eyes the moment I passed over the threshold and he could see open sky. I showed this trick to my husband as I gently swung Jordan over the threshold of the doorframe. His eyes would open, close, open, close, cry, hush, cry, hush. It was pathetically amusing. We nicknamed him "Le Misérable," as it seemed he just didn't want to be here with us under any terms.

Jordan hated the car, which was probably good, as I was so overtired and frazzled; it took five to ten seconds for me to interpret the difference between a red light and a green one. I did discover, one fateful afternoon, that if I kept one hand on his foot, he would feel reassured enough to fall asleep. I drove backcountry roads, where there was no traffic, for hours with my body half turned around toward the back seat. I dreamed of sleep as I watched crops grow and went weekly to my chiropractor's office for adjustments to my exhausted, aching, misaligned body. I went just about anywhere that anyone would have me and my screaming infant, just to keep my sanity in check. I even went to the hospital emergency on two separate occasions. One doctor even held Jordan up eye to eye to her and had a playful talk with him telling him to, "get some sleep and stop harassing your mommy so!" I stood to one side and sobbed uncontrollably. I made all kinds of appointments I didn't really need just to help me get through the day.

On two occasions, I admit to having an impulse to open the bedroom window, wrap Jordan up like a football and fire him, like a quarterback, out into the yard. I then imagined taking a hot bath and slipping into a blissful sleep for days knowing that the crying would have ceased. Thankfully, a spark in my escaping sanity would kick in to stop me.

At six months of age, Jordan's crying began to ease somewhat and he sometimes slept at night for three to four hours at a stretch. I felt like an emotionally wrecked firefighter waiting for the next alarm bell. I was so stressed that I could not tolerate any loud noises or new information of any kind.

My husband would come home from work eager to discuss his day at the office, and I would just stare at him in a daze secretly wishing he would also turn magically into a football. I felt so trapped and forsaken and it seemed no one was able to throw me a line of empathy. As I was disengaging, I began to acknowledge the anger that was pooling at the pit of my being. I continued to do my best to keep it suppressed, however it was becoming an independent agent and occasionally it would burst forth surprising myself and my husband. I started to strategically hang pictures over holes I would punch in the walls.

At 12 months, Jordan had already had two vaccines and if I could have foreseen what was coming after the MMR at 15 months, I would have suspended the scheduled shot long enough to do some additional research. But who could have known what was to come? Our doctors tell us these shots are safer than the alternative so we trust them implicitly.

Jordan received the heavily loaded DPTP and MMR shot three months after his first birthday. Although this is usually administered at one year, the doctor recommended waiting an extra three months because of Jordan's prematurity. Eight weeks later, Jordan began to have increasing bouts of constipation until the condition became chronic. He sometimes would only pass stool once or twice every five to seven days. To our horror, he once went two whole weeks without having a single bowel movement. At this juncture he was constantly leaking brown water from around the blockage.

Over the next two years, my husband and I administered more glycerin suppositories and juvenile enemas than either of us care to recall. Jordan was at the hospital emergency on seven separate occasions, screaming in pain, while they administered milk and molasses enemas. I'll never forget the smell of week-old stool in combination with sweetened dairy milk. On one occasion, he was even put under general anaesthetic to have the impacted stool removed by the surgeon!

I remember sleeping on a cot next to Jordan's hospital bed, while three months pregnant with my second child and thinking what a hellish nightmare we were all living. I literally existed for the emergence of stool from my child's rectum. He and I had spent countless hours sitting in the bathroom, he on the toilet and I on the floor reading stories to him, waiting for that blissful plop.

The head pediatric surgeon at CHEO (Children's Hospital for Eastern Ontario) informed us that Jordan would have to remain on Lansoÿl™, a stool softener, for the remainder of his childhood. This red jelly-like medicine made primarily of mineral oil, worked solely in the large intestine and colon, without leaking into the "gut," to soften the stool and encourage evacuation. "Apparently," he said, "this condition is very common among young boys and there is no identifiable root cause known by the medical establishment." In addition to the stool softener, we also put Jordan on whole organic foods, lots of fiber and plenty of water. The idea was to encourage the failing muscles in his rectum to contract enough to remember what their purpose was. So it seemed our job as Jordan's plumbers was to use these mechanistic tactics to convince the flaccid muscles to squeeze the waste to the surface.

For whatever reason, I was disenchanted with the doctor's prognosis and I embarked on a mission to find the root cause of Jordan's ills. This did not start out as a muscular, plumbing issue; some other diabolical entity was at work and I was finally going to wake from my anaesthetized slumber to find out what that was.

CHAPTER 3

HOMEOPATHY, MAGICAL CURE?

I had heard vague positive things about an ancient healing system called Homeopathy. "Why not?" I thought. "Nothing else is working." I called a local homeopath and learned that she was interested in offering a basic introductory class in my area. If I would gather together seven to nine people in my home, I could host weekly sessions and have my session paid for. So for 10 weeks I learned how to prescribe at a very basic level using homeopathic remedies for acute first aid circumstances. I really had no clue why homeopathic remedies worked, but I did know that they were based on natural substances like minerals, plants and animals. And more importantly, they could do no harm!

It was Dr. Samuel Hahnemann, the 18th-century German physician, who had become disillusioned with the side effects of medical treatments and he first applied "Like Cures Like" to cure malaria. While investigating the properties of cinchona bark (quinine), he took a small dose and discovered that he experienced effects very much like the disease transmitted by an infected mosquito. This method of "proving" substances in a "crude form" would lead him to discover the range of symptoms each substance was capable of causing. His genius led him to dilute the crude matter in water in stages, vigorously shaking the solution as he went. When the "potentized" remedy was fed to a patient with malaria, he was miraculously cured! How could dilute matter become stronger than the patient's disease?

This is so counter intuitive that most people new to homeopathy have some significant challenges wrapping their heads around the concept, myself included. Modern physics will even admit that our seemingly solid bodies are really just dense fields of energy. Barbara Ann Brennan[1] worked as a research scientist at NASA's Goddard Space Flight Center. She trained in the area of Bioenergetics and Core Energetic Therapy at the Institute for Psychophysical Synthesis in Washington, D.C. She has illustrated in her book, *Light Emerging, The Journey of Personal Healing* that in order to stay healthy, we must attempt to surround ourselves with "positive energy." Nature, animals and even food pulse at an energetic frequency beneficial to humanity. She suggests that if we match, or increase, the energetic frequency of what we ingest, we have the power to cure ourselves. She goes on to share her concerns about how our foods are so laden with herbicides and pesticides that the pulse of our foods no longer resonates at the required eight megahertz per minute required by our bodies to remain healthy which seriously compromises our ability to absorb nutrients. She goes on to suggest that foods grown organically are the best option available to us.

We are told that if we pay attention to our regimen by exercising, eating well, drinking enough water, sleeping six to eight hours every night and surrounding ourselves with supportive, loving people we will live longer, healthier lives. But what happens if our systems are continually compromised by stresses, seemingly beyond our control, and we actually incur a chronic condition that won't let up? Sometimes, if we are able to nip it in the bud, quickly paying attention to the issue at hand, we can reverse the "impregnation" of the issue. We stay home from work the next day, drink plenty of fluids and send in regular doses of vitamin C and all seems to have resolved on its own by the next day.

However, what can we do when the issue does "stay for the night?" Impregnation ensues and we know intuitively that no matter how much we exercise, sleep or eat well that we may not be able to halt the condition in its tracks. While it is true that diseases like Aids, Cancer, Hodgkin's, Lupus, or Multiple

Sclerosis can effectively be "managed" through a variety of therapies that keep symptoms at bay, cure through these means is rarer than we would like.

Homeopathy, "homoios" and "pathos" are derived from the Greek, meaning "similar suffering." "Like Cures Like" is based on the fact that a medicinal substance can create a similar, artificial disease in a healthy person. If we ingest a tiny crude dose of chocolate, for example, we can document the effects over minutes and hours. We would be very surprised to see that chocolate can produce symptoms of euphoria in the short term, and then restlessness and low-level anxiety over the next couple of hours.

This process is called a "Proving," and Dr. Hahnemann performed 99 full provings in his lifetime while developing the system of homeopathy. The Law of Similars states that if you derive an energetic dose from the crude matter and feed it back to a patient suffering "chocolate disease," you in effect will cure it! Although counter intuitive to our materialistic minds, the artificially administered disease matter will overshadow the natural disease, thus allowing the organism to free itself from it.

Medicine, like any science, must be firmly based on the actions of nature. Just as gravity dictates what happens if you throw a ball up into the air, natural law must be considered in every pursuit we undertake. If we work in a contrary fashion, we risk a great deal through harming ourselves.

We are conditioned to think that cure is outside the boundaries of possibility. In fact, a system of medicine must be solely based on cure as its premise, as anything else is truly a compromise. If a medicine is prescribed on the basis of principle and natural law, then the result must be permanent and gentle.

As cited by Rudolf Verspoor and Steven Decker[2] in *The Dynamic Legacy: From Homeopathy to Heilkunst*, the first aim of medicine is to prevent disease, but once disease has taken hold of a person, then the aim must be to destroy it, ultimately effecting cure. No other standard will do!

Since Hippocrates' time, individuals have been attempting to discover the laws of nature and how we might use them for our benefit. Science was referred to as natural philosophy, or the rational study of nature. The roots of western medicine stem from the observations of nature by Greek philosophers several thousand years ago. In fact, during the "Golden Age of Greece," the Greeks were the ones to draw rational conclusions from the systematic study of nature. This is where rational conclusions were first formulated in the form of hypotheses, theories, laws and principles.

Out of these Greek writings, two principles of nature were consciously applied to medicine: the law of similars and the law of opposites. In other words, medicinal therapeutics can either work on the basis of producing a similar action on a patient with a natural disease (homeopathic), or produce an opposite action to that of the disease (antipathic). Where there is no conscious natural principle, but only blind effect is intended we have allopathic medicine. The law of similars cures in disease, whereas the law of opposites removes imbalances, such as in nutrition.

When I was just learning the basics of homeopathy, for example, Jordan developed a sudden high fever. I was awakened by his screams in the middle of the night and I tore out of bed and down the hall to his room. When I reached for him the night light illumined his very red face and ears. His head was burning, his eyes glistened dizzily and as the panic ascended my spine, I noticed his pupils were dilated. As I stared at him blankly, wondering what to do, I carried him to the medicine chest. Behind the glass, stood the usual over-the-counter pain relief medications and the few homeopathic remedies I had acquired recently. Taking his temperature seemed like a logical thing to do as I considered our options. As I stuck the electronic device into his armpit, I wondered if I had learned enough about homeopathy to hazard a guess at what to prescribe in this case? Jordan's fever was a whopping 104.5 degrees Fahrenheit!

I took out my book on homeopathic medicine for children as he alternated cries and murmurings and I held his feverish body in my arms. The remedy *Belladonna* seemed to be the "similimum" I was searching for and I happened to have a low potency in my burgeoning pharmacy. I dropped a couple of the little white pellets into his mouth and waited. He seemed to settle and I lay down beside him and skeptically waited for him to cry out again so that I could give him the dose of acetaminophen as usual. The latter always seemed to work.

Jordan and I slept in late that morning, and when he finally woke, it was as if nothing had taken place during the night. His fever was completely gone and there was no redness in his cheeks. Although the bed sheets were damp, I wondered if I had imagined the whole scene, except that I was sleeping in his bed. A sure sign something had transpired!

I realized much later when studying to be a physician of homeopathy that I had in fact followed the law of similars in that instance and prescribed a medicine that in fact produced a similar state of fever in Jordan. It in effect cancelled out the first, natural disease, producing a seemingly magical cure.

If I had chosen the acetaminophen, as I had done in the past, I would have been in the realm of "Allopathy" which is defined as the use of a medicine against disease in the form of "contraries" and at best could only have provided temporary relief. By suppressing the fever, I could have potentially blocked the natural avenues of healing caused by the inflammation.

The latter move in effect short-circuits the body's ability to "close the loop" on the disease at hand. In essence, the life force will become frustrated in its attempts and will find other ways to express what it needs for its ultimate evolution. Through the vaccination of childhood diseases we are effectively compromising our children's proper immune functioning. By applying the law of similars to disease, you are following the direction of cure naturally. When the heat-seeking missile hits the target, the person's condition starts to improve. For example, you will remember that Jordan quieted after receiving the remedy *Belladonna* and he was able to return to sleep. Other things you may notice is that the person seems to relax, achieving "a greater degree of comfort, increasing composure, freedom of spirit, increased courage – a kind of returning to naturalness."[3] The other thing to be aware of is that the direction of cure occurs from the inside to the outside. If I had been able to stay awake that night, and watched Jordan after he had fallen back to sleep, I might have witnessed the fever descend and a sweat break out on his skin.

Dr. Hahnemann refers to the body's organs in an order of hierarchy; the skin obviously being the most external and one of the least noble organs of the body. The body is designed to push disease out to the least noble organs in order to preserve the core where the more noble organs reside. However, the opposite can be true when disease is suppressed by drugs. The disease will just be driven further into the core of the being. Our bodies are designed very much like a merry-go-round. Centrifugal force will always try to force disease out to the surface. Our sweat, mucus and urine are purveyors of inimical microbes. You would not consider retaining your urine indefinitely, so why would you choose to carry your symptoms and diseases indefinitely?

I know a woman who used to suffer with severe eczema as a child. She went to her family doctor who prescribed a cortisone cream, the external condition seemed to clear up and she was quite happy with the results. That autumn, she noticed that she developed hay fever and asthma. She returned to the doctor to see what could be done and she left with a prescription for a "puffer," also containing cortisone. Her hay fever seemed to diminish, providing she kept on using the drug. However, she noticed that she was feeling more and more depressed. When I met her, she was using prednisone for this condition and she wanted to get off all the drugs as she was suffering from a variety of side effects including damage to her liver.

My understanding of the effects of homeopathy were really borne out of a skepticism that cure was actually tangible, available and attainable. On top of that, I also felt that it should be a struggle, invasive and difficult! As I think back on that moment when I was transitioning my thinking, I began to feel so incredibly empowered that I could affect cure easily without any further harm. It was monumental to me that if my child was stung by a bee, sunburned or developed an ear infection, I could address the issue safely and effectively right there at home. In those early days, it began to mean even more to me that, not only could I save an already burdened health care system another trip or two to the family doctor, I could actually restore health.

My level of fear also went down a peg or two and I worried less when we took trips camping or hiking where the potential for injury in a remote area was greater. It meant that I took my own personal jurisdiction of healing up a notch and I read everything on homeopathy I could get my hands on. Jordan and I started spending a lot more time at the local library in the section under alternative therapies. I was gaining an ounce more freedom, page-by-page, and experience-by-experience.

CHAPTER 4

BAD BOY BEHAVIOUR

At the age of three, Jordan's chief problems were chronic constipation and very profound behavioural issues. Often he would not pass stool for a week or more. This was alarming enough on its own, but the toxicity stored in his body produced conduct resembling what traditional medicine was calling Attention Deficit Hyperactivity Disorder, or ADHD. He could not focus for a minute on any one activity. There was a violent side to him too. He would often haul off and slap me across the face or punch me in the stomach without a moment's notice and with a vindictiveness that astounded me. Waking from afternoon naps, he would often scream for two hours solid while rocking and banging his head against his bedroom wall.

If I reached to console him, he would flail his arms attacking me, so I ran around the house like a crazed firefighter searching for a cure. I would try to get him to sniff an open jar of coffee or I would try to pop a homeopathic pellet of *Chamomilla* into his mouth in an effort to calm him. I usually ended up with coffee grounds all through the carpet. Now that I think about it, smelling the coffee would have been an attempt to match his emotional state of mind homeopathically. Like might have cured like if the dose was the simillimum and energetically strong enough!

However, Jordan wasn't having anything to do with any principled approach and these bouts of anger were becoming more eruptive. I felt I was always on heightened alert to diffuse potential barriers or triggers that would set off an exaggerated response. If I missed the opportunity, the screaming and flailing could last for hours. I was failing miserably at predicting the future and becoming a hopelessly neurotic firefighter.

Family members accused me of not being firm enough and they went as far as to comment that Jordan was, "obviously in charge of the parents as opposed to the other way around." Even though these comments hurt to my very core, I secretly agreed with them. But I was so exhausted and lost in the magnitude of our situation that I just could not fully comprehend the nightmare that had become my day-to-day existence. Any sense of me as an individual woman, let alone a wife or mother, was lost in the minute-to-minute triage that defined my existence with Jordan.

I'm not sure I had a very well-defined ego going into marriage and childbirth, however, any semblance of this "body" had been effectively lost during this day-to-day inferno of anguish. If I left the room to use the washroom, Jordan would let out the most blood-curdling scream that I just took him with me everywhere, 24 hours a day, seven days a week, and 365 days of the year.

Assuming Jordan was expressing issues of abandonment I had created shortly after his birth, I made it my personal mission to help fill these vacuous holes in my beloved son's psyche. As I look back, my assumption was based on what I desperately needed and craved myself. The efforts I made were really about me trying to fill my own personal wantonness since my mother had abandoned me. "Oh, what a tangled web we weave, when we practise to deceive (our inner child) …"

As a result, I had effectively created a situation where I had no reprieve except when my husband came home to lend a hand or my mother-in-law came in from out of town. She put Jordan in his carriage and walked around the neighbourhood for hours. During that precious time, I watched out the window with a constant low level anxiety and attempted to recall the semblance of my self.

Too wired with stress to take a nap, I would try to sit quietly with my eyes closed, sensing my own breath. Air swept past nostril hairs, cooling my throat, expanding my chest and returning out the same passage, only warm now and full of moisture, holding the tears I held deeply inside.

On the couch in the basement family room, my husband would often rest with Jordan lying against his bare chest so that I could sleep late on the occasional weekend morning. They would both be covered with a thick blanket and Jordan would settle into a deep sleep provided he was hot enough to be dripping with sweat, with his ear on his dad's beating heart.

I secretly wished for that cocoon-like surrender to warmth and nurturing. I was so frazzled, I was sure I was worsening Jordan's condition. I added buckets of guilt to my already beleaguered psyche. What was one more bucketful of unresolved angst?

CHAPTER 5

JORDAN MEETS HOMEOPATHY

I began to take Jordan regularly to my chiropractor who gently held pressure points on his body to help release the emotional and physical toxicity that was stored there. This helped to a degree, in the short-term, but it was as if Jordan's body had a "muscular and skeletal memory" of the underlying rooted conditions and everything would be pulled back into its original position once we left the office. We could address a subluxation or two on the surface, but the root cause continued to mock us from the core of his little being.

I was regularly ordering remedies from a local homeopathic dispensary and I became quite friendly with the owner as I continued to prescribe acutely for my family. I liked her and I probed whether she provided consultations for more chronic conditions as I explained to her the issues that plagued Jordan. She said that she did this on occasion and we set up an appointment.

She used remedies that I was not familiar with. She prescribed low potencies of *Thuja Occidentalis, Psorinum, Tuberculinum, Medorrhinum,* and *Syphilinum* taken one at a time and waiting a couple of weeks in between. I was also instructed that Jordan should abstain from taking any other remedies in order to avoid short-circuiting the effects of one remedy with another. I wondered what would happen if he cut himself and needed *Calendula* during this treatment. Did this mean that I could potentially disrupt the action of one remedy by introducing another? When I asked her this, she answered that this was indeed the case. Intuitively, I was uneasy about her answer. On several occasions in the past, I had administered a number of remedies at one time. When my daughter had fallen and hit her head, I had given her *Natrum Sulphuricum* for potential concussion after a head injury, *Arnica* for bruising, and *Hypericum* for any nerve damage. There didn't appear to be any negative repercussions or ill effects and it seemed that the injuries had been cured just the same. I chose to use my discretion in this regard.

I followed the instructions as closely as was reasonable and waited and watched to see what clues of a cure would unfold. Jordan's behaviour and constipation improved a little at first, but then seemed to get much worse than before taking the remedies. The homeopath felt that this was normal and in fact a good sign that we had the right remedy. Like a slingshot, with homeopathy there is often a pulling back into illness before projecting forward into healing. Finally, after a subsequent treatment, Jordan improved quite markedly for a couple of weeks. But then, sadly, his symptoms returned.

The homeopath reminded me that since there had been some improvement, we were on the right track, and she attempted to repeat the exact same prescription of remedy and dose. Again, we saw improvement, but for a shorter time than the last, before his return to the original state. The cause and treatment of Jordan's problems still eluded us.

This dance was very similar to what we experienced at the chiropractor's office. I remember feeling quite frustrated with the whole state of affairs. I had briefly tasted freedom for Jordan, and saw my little boy in a state of grace for a short while. I wanted more and was determined that the answer lay somewhere within the scope of this ancient medical system. I went to the library and ordered every book I could find on homeopathy. Perhaps Jordan's homeopath was somehow underutilizing the system.

At our next visit, when I suggested some alternate remedies like *Alumina*, she clearly became defensive and I realized that she was not at all on sure ground with my son's chronic issues. When she asked me how his progress had been in the last month, I confessed that I had felt the need to intervene with some other remedies I had been exploring in the *Homeopathic Materia Medicas* I had researched. She reacted rather angrily and accused me of not supporting her efforts to help my son. She told me unequivocally that she would now have to utilize the same remedies I had administered "in error" in order to reverse all the potential damage I had done to his treatment.

That was the last time I took Jordan to see her for any of his chronic complaints. This was one of the most ridiculous declarations I had heard since first being exposed to this esoteric art. Did she mean to tell me that the body could only manage one informed remedy at a time? Why couldn't energy separate each issue to treat six problems at once, for example? I couldn't find anyone with the homeopathic "Rule Book!"

In essence, because there was no material dose in the potencies I had used, how did she intend to harness the animated principle and reverse it? I had learned that if a remedy was not required by the body, then it would just find a way out through urine, sweat or mucus membranes without harm to the patient. I went home to ruminate over what had transpired and re-evaluate what I had learned about homeopathy so far. As I headed back to the library to wade through more material, I acknowledged that I felt isolated and alone. Medically, I was at a dead end and I found myself on my own again.

CHAPTER 6

JORDAN'S FINAL EFFORT TO "HANG ON"

A friend of mine suggested I take Jordan to see another homeopath who practised a different approach to homeopathy. I was fairly skeptical by this time and I shook off her suggestion until my step-mother, who coincidently was also studying homeopathy at the time, fortuitously switched to study with a new school where a new system of thought was championed. I knew based on my limited knowledge, that I was in no position to treat Jordan's chronic issues myself, so I made an appointment at the Hahnemann Center for Heilkunst Clinic about five minutes from my home.

The week before Jordan's appointment with the homeopathic physician, Patty Smith, also Dean of Student Affairs of The Hahnemann College for Heilkunst, we found ourselves back in a crisis with very impacted stool and another hospital visit looming. Patty encouraged me to come to her home to pick up a homeopathic remedy to try to address Jordan's immediate needs.

Both of Patty's enthusiastic daughters met us at their front door with domestic rats in hand. At the age of four, Jordan found this a rare treat and enjoyed a few moments molesting the well-loved rodents. Patty and I chatted about Jordan's condition and she handed me a little brown dropper bottle with a label and some writing on it. At a glance, I was surprised to see that there were a number of remedies, including *Alumina*, contained in the one bottle. I did not recognize most of them and the potencies were higher than what I, and the previous homeopath, were accustomed to using. The contents appeared as innocuous as water, and Patty suggested I put a drop in Jordan's water and let him sip on it throughout the day until the stubborn stool emerged. I was very hopeful.

By the next morning, Jordan still had not emitted the eagerly awaited deliverance and we got in the car to head to Toronto over Thanksgiving for a Jewish holiday. As usual, there were many family events to celebrate and by Saturday Jordan was leaking runny brown water from around the impacted stool. Sadly, at age four, he still wore "pull-on" diapers for this reason.

Typically, he would run to the corner of a room, fixate on something, stand on his toes and squeeze his bum cheeks together with all his might. Every muscle in his body tensed toward his mission to maintain control. This was the stance he invariably assumed every time his body would attempt to emit the toxic stool he held within.

This campaign against the emergence of his excrement had gone on solidly for two and a half years. I can't even begin to count the number of times I had gently encouraged him by saying, "Try to relax and let go!" It appeared as if he was hanging on with every fiber of his being. This always astounded my husband and me. The counterproductive quality of his condition seemed to go completely against the laws of nature.

Later on, during my research into this fairly common condition that apparently often plagues boys in early childhood, this precise stance was described by many parents and we all agreed how astoundingly detrimental to the intended outcome it seemed. What imaginable reason provoked these little men to hold on to their stool for days and even weeks at a time? I know that I am much closer to knowing the answer to this question today.

We ended up leaving the family gathering to take Jordan to the local hospital for yet another enema. We were worn out, disillusioned and exasperated with the same scenario beating at our consciousness and I once again felt my hopes dashed where homeopathy was concerned. Why couldn't we help Jordan with a seemingly inane function like passing his own stool? My husband and I felt that we had more than failed him with our inability to grasp the root cause of his ills.

After a torturous two hours of attempting to hold in the effects of two adult enemas, Jordan passed a large, but very soft stool from his rectum. I noted this in the recesses of my psyche as he fell asleep, exhausted, in my arms. We took our sweet warrior back to his grandparents for the night. Unbeknownst to us, this would be the last hospital visit Jordan would have to endure for this chronic complaint.

CHAPTER 7

SEQUENTIAL THERAPY?

Patty Smith's office was located in a beautiful stone century home just east of Ottawa, Ontario. I felt an assured calm the moment we crossed the threshold. My step-mom had offered to come with us in case I needed help keeping Jordan entertained so that I could focus on what Patty was saying. Naturally, my step-mom was also eager to learn how to address his condition from a clinical standpoint, as she was in the throes of her studies in homeopathy at Patty and Rudolf Verspoor's International School, The Hahnemann College for Heilkunst. Patty and Rudi are actually married and they dedicate their lives to furthering this particular art of medicine.

Patty began to describe Heilkunst as a system of medicine based on Dr. Hahnemann's complete writings that takes traditional, the more conventional or "classical" homeopathy to a whole new level. From what I could tell, the remedies were just a part of a whole approach to lift all of the physical and emotional shocks Jordan had sustained since birth. As I explained our prior experience with the other classical homeopath, Patty told me that this is very common as the remedies were being prescribed based on symptoms alone as opposed to cause. Also, classical homeopathy interpreted Hahnemann to say one remedy per person as opposed to one remedy per disease. A Heilkünstler will treat for all concordant disease simultaneously.

It was also first explained to me that when Dr. Samuel Hahnemann's body of work entitled the *Organon der Heilkunst* was translated into English, a very important discernment between imbalance and disease was overlooked, as well as a fundamental distinction between primary diseases and secondary diseases. The physicians attempting to interpret his work at the time mistakenly reported the two sides of disease as being the same thing.

It was Patty's husband, Rudolf Verspoor, educated to use the classical approach, who began to question certain limitations during his own treatment. He was also at a real crossroad with a few of his own patients who were just not getting any better. Rudi tells the story of how, during a layover in an airport he happened upon a book entitled *Rediscovering Real Medicine*, authored by the Swiss doctor, Dr. Jean Elmiger.[4] Although he struggled in his efforts to comprehend the deeper aspects of the original French, suddenly an electrical current seemed to connect the dots in his mind. If the writing was correct, homeopathy had been underutilized for the last two hundred years!

Dr. Elmiger saw that we are animated by the law of bipolarity, the Yin and the Yang so to speak. He illustrates this phenomenon very simply by describing his simple desk lamp, "with only one wire, the electrical current could not produce light." Our bodies are mapped out the same way energetically and Elmiger determined that treatment should address life's shocks and traumas as they are retained by the body in our cellular memory over the course of our lifetimes. In essence, the more shocks and traumas we sustain, the further apart our polarity spans, and the more out of balance we become.

Elmiger realized that our life represents one long series of energetic disturbances. The one side of us that sustains our health will signal to us through the use of symptoms, a runny nose or sore throat for example. This sustaining side can stabilize and rebalance after receiving one or two shocks, especially if there are long periods of calm and repose in between.

However, later, when Rudi partnered with Steven Decker, scholar par excellence of the German and the Romantic Thought Movement, they saw very clearly that it was Dr. Samuel Hahnemann who had actually first seen the two sides of the living principle and disease. As Steven was translating the sixth edition of Hahnemann's *Organon of the Medical Art*, he in effect unearthed the simple, but dynamic multi-dimensional system of medicine that respects two sides of disease. To this day, no other system of medicine recognizes the implications of Hahnemann's true genius.

While Rudi was exploring the possibility that something was missing in his own approach from a clinical standpoint, Steven was unearthing this dual system for cure in his intellectual research. Both met through a series of coincidental events at Steven's house in California.

Incidentally, both Steven and Rudi are born on the same day, a couple of years apart; both look very similar in that they are tall, slim and have a healthy shock of silver hair. Witnessing them lecturing together is a little like watching the dual nature of a very animated and brilliant comedy team; reading their works is like being exposed to history and principle as you have never seen it illumined before. Their body of collaborative work entitled *Dynamic Legacy: From Homeopathy to Heilkunst* is rendered in a surprisingly simple and shockingly brilliant way.

Both Rudi and Steven are from the opposite end of the spectrum of constitutions. While this will be illustrated more clearly later, Rudi is *Silicea*, which means that he formulates his thoughts using a more cosmic, bridled, spherical influence which is easy to interpret. Steven is *Sulphur*, which means that he derives his way of thinking from the thrusty energy of the earth pole. He has a much larger presence and conveys his thoughts much more flamboyantly. In essence, the dual nature of disease and the living principle, the intrinsic element to cure, was being reborn in the new millennium by two very opposite individuals. The yin and the yang in motion!

How is seeing this dual nature so critical you ask? Well, all forms of medicine and those practising homeopathy since Hahnemann's day over the last 200 years have only seen the *sustaining side* of our living principle. The realm of *imbalance*! Every day, we sustain ourselves by drinking, eating, sleeping, voiding and moving.

Imagine that you awaken one morning with a sore throat, the inability to swallow easily, a heavy head and are a little warm to the touch. You may take a couple of vitamin "Cs", call in to work letting them know that you are staying home to rest that day and crawl back into bed and sleep for a few more hours. You may reawaken feeling better. After a couple bowls of chicken soup and another good night's rest, you may be 99 percent better and ready to re-engage in your life.

In essence, you used your sustaining energy, or *Sustentive* power, to make the necessary corrections to get better. The illness was just a superficial call for rest and remediation that did not require medicine. In fact, there was no disease present at all.

Traditional chiropractic, massage therapy, the health food and vitamin industry, and even allopathic (traditional Western) medicine are examples of approaches built primarily on restoring imbalance by suppressing or at best palliating the Sustentive side of the living power. Their approach is based on giving more or taking away what is too little or too much. If there is a Vitamin C deficiency, you give more Vitamin C. If the heart doesn't beat regularly enough, you install a pacemaker. For a sore neck, give a massage or a chiropractic adjustment. They focus on correcting the imbalance, assuming that this will cure the disease.

Now, if we back up for a moment and put you back in bed with the sore throat and the fever rising, you may have felt congestion descending into your chest and a loud hard cough may have kept you up most of the next night. You know that at a minimum you won't be going into work the next day. After a couple of days of sleeplessness, racking cough and misery, you know that you have incurred something that a couple of Vitamin Cs and a pot of chicken soup is not going to be able to lick on its own. Now, disease has affected the Generative side of the living power and a true reversal would require the Law of Similars.

In effect, disease is beyond the realm of imbalance. The Generative is all about being dynamically affected and impregnated by disease. It has the power to seduce and alter your life force through energetic resonance and it is not leaving until it has had its way with you. You might want to set another chair at the table, because the disease will be staying for breakfast.

And this isn't the "dis-ease" that affects your vitality that the doctor, chiropractor and health food store operator refer to.

Disease affecting the Generative is constant, chronic, and as mentioned before, can only be cured one way, using the Law of Similars. For example recurring bronchitis is often anchored to tuberculosis, recurring moles can be anchored to cancer, and chronic hand washing can be anchored to syphilis. You can take antibiotics, have the moles removed or send the patient to the psychiatrist, but you will not affect the chronic constant disease that remains anchored to the Generative.

However, this is typically the point at which you cart yourself off to the doctor. A swab of your yellow-green sputum may be sent off to the lab for analysis, a diagnosis of "bronchitis" is rendered and you may go home with a prescription for antibiotics just like last winter and the winter before that. In the short term, you seemed to get better and you took some acidophilus and bifidus in an effort to replenish the good bacteria to rebuild your immunity. What you may not be aware of, however, is that by short-circuiting the body's inflammatory process, there may be a further price to pay down the line.

The word "anti" means "against or opposing"; "bios" means "a way of life"; so "antibiotics" means "destroying life or preventing the inception or continuance of life." When we take antibiotics, our body does not tell the antibiotics which specific microbes to annihilate. They, in effect, waltz in and indiscriminately wipe out both "bad" and "good" bacteria. This avenue of treatment short-circuits the inflammatory response of the body, which is really an indication of the Sustentive power rallying to fight off the "disease" in its efforts to restore balance. If the Sustentive power is allowed to do its job, you may get better in a few more days of rest with plenty of fluids. The fever may even get quite high in its efforts to burn off the negative microbial agents, and if allowed to finish the job, it will usually heal you in a day or so. After letting your body fight it off on its own, you may feel even stronger and better than you did before you got sick. Your immune system may even improve and your vitality may be greater than before.

Children will often experience a healthy growth spurt after having the chicken pox, provided that there was no interference from chemical drug therapy. Researchers are now linking diseases such as cancer and even HIV as the long-term effects of continuing to eliminate our childhood illnesses. Indeed, we are effectively compromising the Generative power by not trusting our body's wisdom.

Referring again to the eczema example mentioned earlier, the allopathic doctor may prescribe a cortisone cream, which may or may not clear up the problem on the surface. However, next spring, the patient begins to suffer with airborne allergies. The patient returns to the doctor who now prescribes a cortisone-based puffer that she inhales regularly during the month of May every year. Not surprisingly, the following year, she may now be suffering with low-level depression and wonders, "why now," when she never felt this way in her life before. Suppression in effect has pushed the disease into her core one level at a time.

In essence, this common scenario is contrary to the direction of cure, which should be from "the inside out." If you go back to the example of the Merry-Go-Round, our bodies are designed to eliminate toxicity and disease using centrifugal force. We would not think to hold in our sweat, mucus, urine and feces indefinitely, so why would we want to do the same with the symptoms of disease? By suppressing the symptoms, we drive the disease deeper each time we use chemical drugs. Unfortunately, there are no exceptions to this rule. This is the law of cure. From the inside out is the only way to true health.

So let's continue with another scenario. Let's say you are back in bed, again, and after five days, you are not getting any better. Things are even more distraught, you're alone in a cabin in the middle of Antarctica and you are also suffering hypothermia. Sadly, you are becoming increasingly weaker from being cold, you are coughing, and past delirious from fever and blood has been showing up in your sputum for days. You are in dire straits. You could soon lose consciousness and even die.

In this scenario, the life force is designed to "offer up" body parts in a certain order in an attempt to save the core. It does a tally of the noblest organs in an effort to provoke the Sustentive into healing itself. Gangrene is an example of this functioning. You never hear of someone getting gangrene of the heart and having to cut it out to save the leg! Fever works the same way. It attempts to "cook" the microbes and push them out to the surface through sweat, urine and mucus. It is important to note that once the Generative is affected by disease, there is only one path to cure. The principled Law of Cure is based on Like Cures Like and there is no other way!

So let me tie up all these loose ends by giving you an example. Jordan was born in July and every winter for his first two years of life, when he cut a tooth, he would start by getting a cold, his ears would become infected and then he would develop bronchitis and then pneumonia. He cycled through this pattern two to three times per winter. I took him to the doctor, the same diagnosis was rendered and the prescription for antibiotics was administered.

Jordan's infections became increasingly worse after each bout and he was not gaining any weight. In addition, he was only passing stool once every one to two weeks. I knew that his health was slowly being destroyed and I felt powerless to do anything.

We were attempting to address his symptoms repeatedly with the same therapeutic approach, while the root of the issue was just waiting for the opportunity to re-manifest. In essence, stool softener, increased water intake, vitamin therapy, regular chiropractic care and organic foods were not having the desired impact on his stool impaction. This approach to therapy was also difficult to manage with a three year old, and I always felt I was on a tightrope verging on the next tragic fall. He would toss his food across the room as his behaviour spiralled out of control.

When Jordan began Heilkunst treatment, Patty asked me to write out his timeline. I had to list all of his life traumas, in reverse order, from today back to his birth. Traumas were any events, large or small, that could have impacted his physical, emotional, mental or spiritual well-being. These events included our various trips to the hospital, colds, ear infections, any separations from me or his father, falls, sunburn—anything! Heilkunst treatment uses homeopathic remedies to reverse each of these traumas, effectively peeling off the layers of trauma one by one, leaving a healthy, whole person.

We could quickly see how each event peppered Jordan's timeline creating the boy we had come to know, eclipsed by disease. His timeline indicated traumas sustained at the hospital emergency with the milk and molasses enemas, and the countless pediatric enemas at home. We had used numerous boxes of glycerin suppositories and I was very concerned about how these invasive treatments had affected him emotionally more than physically. The timeline showed rounds of antibiotics from bouts of ear infections and pneumonia over the first two winters of his life and a fall from a play structure at the local park where he sustained a bruise or two, and the time when he fell out of bed and broke his collarbone. Then his timeline showed all his vaccinations, not to mention the stress of his prematurity and birth. No wonder he was so angry!

Patty used homeopathic remedies to treat Jordan's physical and emotional symptoms. These included remedies for anger, grief, envy, fear and anxiety. These were put into a little brown dropper bottle with some distilled water. She also gave us a dropper for his constipation as well as "tonic" remedies to sequentially strip off the effects of the enemas and suppositories, rounds of antibiotics, the vaccination shocks and his birth trauma.

Patty was treating both sides of Jordan's disease simultaneously – the symptoms being expressed by the Sustentive power and the underlying hidden or "tonic" diseases. The real healing came from the latter. Jordan began to heal. Because of the remedies, his body began to generate what it needed to resolve what was energetically outstanding. His generative side woke up. I saw my son getting profoundly better, quickly, and without chemical intervention. By nailing the underlying causes, balance was being restored and the symptoms were disappearing. Finally, no more tightrope walking and no more firefighting, a semblance of peace at last! Thank God.

Jordan got significantly better after treatment for his vaccination shocks and we eventually achieved complete and lasting cure of his entire lung and constipation complaints. This involved another level of timeline therapy, treating the chronic miasms.

The chronic miasms are the genetic or inherited diseases which are at the root of most chronic illness. Somewhere in my husband's or my genetic make-up was the significant predisposition for bronchial infections and it was not going anywhere until annihilated using timeline therapy and the law of similars. Jordan is nine and a half now, and has not had one bout of pneumonia since those first two years. He spent so much time being sick as an infant and toddler that he had an enormous amount of living to catch up on. We were finally freed from the burden of managing his chronic complaints.

We also watched the uprooting of a number of other issues related to the other chronic miasms that danced down our family lines. I could not believe that his chronic diaper rash cleared during the treatment called *Medhorrinum* and the last threads of his behaviour disorders lifted during *Syphilinum* treatment. From my perspective these were just gravy on Jordan's plate of cure as the conditions we originally sought help for were long gone.

When shocks persist over a person's lifetime, they increase the potential for more resonant impregnation of the person's life force on the level of the generative and prevent the Sustentive element from doing its job effectively. As Hahnemann said, it is one big job to keep all parts of our organism in "admirable, harmonious, vital operation, regulating both our feelings and functions, so that our spirit can freely avail itself of the healthy, higher purposes of our existence."[5] For me, this 200-year-old statement is the absolute key to why Heilkunst treatment is so critical. Through this process we had given Jordan the gift of his life to be lived the way he always desired it, unencumbered and free.

Our life force is like a snowball heading down the slope of life. A car accident where you sustained injuries may cause you to pick up some small rocks as you continue down the mountain. You are still rolling in the right direction. However, there is now a noticeable wobble and your balance is off. You are moving slower and veering to the right. Antibiotic use may be compared to rolling over a stick or two, causing further hindrance to the smooth roll of the ball. With the death of a family member, the ball becomes weighed down with a very large rock. As you experience further shocks and traumas, things can really start to get off kilter and the ball may start heading for a cliff. Now would be a good time to intervene.

If medicine is to move forward, then it is critical for us to acknowledge that when chronic illness has the opportunity to impregnate the Generative side of the life force, any number of attempts to "rebalance" will not work. As you can see, no vitamin, herb or drug therapy is effectively going to address the root cause of disease when it hits this side of the life force. Symptom upon symptom will have the opportunity to anchor from the impregnated root on the Generative side and there is only one principled law of nature that can cure it, the law of similars.

In the early days, Rudi broadened his approach to include Dr. Elmiger's sequential treatment using the homeopathic remedies to effectively remove one shock or trauma at a time. As he began to treat his patients like an onion using this form of therapy, stripping off one event on their timeline after another, he noticed that the symptoms were disappearing permanently. The anchor to which they were rooted was effectively ripped up and permanently annihilated.

While sequential treatment was becoming one of the cornerstones of Rudi's approach with his patients, he still searched for explanations and guiding principles for this system of medicine. Steven Decker was aware of the two sides of the living principle, but was unsure how it would look if applied clinically. I would have loved to have been in that hotel room when the two sides of disease were first discussed by the scholar and confirmed by the clinician. History was remade after sleeping for 200 years. Certainly, a Dynamic Legacy!

CHAPTER 8

BACK TO JORDAN

From that first visit to Patty's, Jordan's behaviour was remarkable during consultations and he always played beautifully by himself. I even thought that she might not believe all of what I had to tell her regarding his violent behaviour. I remember being struck by a moment while he was occupied with the blocks and thinking how awesome he was and how much he was going to teach me. He suddenly looked up at me and smiled so knowingly, I felt taken out of the moment and to a place of realization. It was almost as if he looked at me to say, "I was wondering how long it would take before you brought us here!"

I felt in that moment that Jordan knew where we were and why. That it was somehow predestined and I was just fulfilling an intended role in his life. The outcome was written and it was up to me to just participate and trust. I knew I could let go, and I didn't have to will him better anymore all by myself.

At the end of the session, Patty gave us a warm hug good-bye and we went off with two little dropper bottles for Jordan's emotional issues and a little coin envelope with two powder remedies for his most recent timeline event, which was the latest surgery to remove the impacted stool.

After one additional follow-up visit with Patty in December, Jordan was starting to pass stool a little more consistently. Although we had not covered more than two recent events on his timeline, he was doing better solely on the remedies used in the emotional dropper bottle. It was amazing to me to realize that a bottle containing grief, anger, fear and guilt could start things moving for him. Could it really be that a large part of his issues were derived from the emotional realm and not the physical? That thought floored me.

By mid-January I wrote the following e-mail to Patty just after our third consultation with her:

> Hi Patty, I hope you and your family had a great holiday and you're settled into your new home. We certainly have experienced the most extreme homeopathic aggravations in the history of our household. On the tenth day, after the last timeline remedy administered for Jordan's bouts with ear infections and pneumonia, he was experiencing such violent tendencies that I could not let him near his baby sister. His anger and defiance was so extreme, even with doses of the anger remedy from the dropper bottle that I was continually administering, I felt at my wit's end at how to cope should his behaviour continue. I really felt I had experienced the worse case of "ADHD" as he flung himself from furniture to floor striking out, without conscience, at anything and anyone in his path.
>
> Also Jordan had begun to show signs of constipation again as he had in the past (he went six days before I treated him with a Pediatric Fleet Enema), and three days prior I used the combination dropper remedy to attempt to get things moving as recommended in the past, but nothing was seemingly addressing the issue. What was so interesting to me was that he assumed the tightened, rigid "squeeze the bum cheeks stance" he hasn't used for almost two months, now, and he said that he was afraid it would be painful to pass the "poo" on the toilet as it was when he had gone to the hospital. I offered that he could pass the stool in a pair of pull-on diapers if it made him more comfortable and he has chosen that means since he passed the large plug yesterday morning. He now has a very soft stool resembling mashed potatoes

which he has not had since he was nursed. It feels as if he is cleansing more at an emotional level rather than just the physical.

The next morning, Jordan woke on New Year's Day with a sunny disposition, and he asked me, "how I was doing?" I almost fell over as in all his four years, he had never engaged me in such a way and I wasn't sure how to answer him as I hadn't taken the time to ask myself that question in years. He was ecstatic at the possibility of spending the day at the indoor swimming pool. The day before, it would have angered him to no end if we had made any decisions around anything that affected him.

Since the New Year, he has been very affectionate saying how much he loves each one of us and wanting to be held many times throughout the day. I can't believe it is him as he crosses the room with his arms open wide. He has also exhibited a desire to play by himself for the first time in his life as well as a friendly desire to be included without demanding that his needs be met in an angry fashion which has been so typical to date. He is also much more inquisitive and we are thrilled to answer his questions until he is satiated.

I know that we probably still have a rough road ahead, but I can tell you, Patty, it is these brief glimpses that make me feel like we are on the right path. Maybe you can give me some constructive tools to handle some of these bouts of anger, as they take such a toll on all our abilities to cope. Also, I read Sam's case from your school's internet site. Rick and I clung to every word as it helps to maintain our focus and hope to see that other families have endured a lot of the same internal angst we have, and survived, to see their son cured.

It is also of great importance to note that Jordan had gained a much needed five pounds since Thanksgiving and he was now eating more varieties of foods including vegetables and tiny bits of meat, which he could not tolerate previously. His water consumption had improved to almost five glasses per day. He had not eaten more than three to four bites of a very bland food per sitting up until now and he had not gained five pounds in over a year and a half.

Over the next ten months Jordan would continue his leaps and bounds towards health and balance. By the third month after his initial consultation, he was running to the bathroom and closing the door to simply "go poo."

I remember one of the first days, I was right behind him as he had run in from playing outside, and I just assumed that he would want me with him in the bathroom as usual. The door closed in my face and I could hear his pants hitting the floor on the other side of the barrier. He emitted a couple of grunts and then the toilet water echoed back his successful efforts with two resounding splashes.

I remember sliding down the other side of that door to sit and stare at the mirror of the closet door before me. I stared at my reflection, the woman before me barely recognizable. The tears flowed from my eyes as I cradled my head in my hands and wept with joy with the realization that we had actually arrived. We were here.

That day marked the first in Jordan's new quality of life, which to me was as tangible as the first day I held my baby rabbit. I continued to sob floods of relieved and exalted tears. I was brought to my senses when he yelled out with a singsong cadence, "Come and wipe my bum!" I thought at that moment that I would be happy to wipe his bum until his first date if he liked!

That first year, Jordan gained 12 pounds and two and a half shoe sizes, and his dances into the realm of "ADHD-like" behaviour lessened month by month as we addressed his timeline trauma by trauma. By watching where his most profound healing reactions were and noting where the biggest improvements manifested, we learned that Jordan's issues were primarily anchored in his vaccinations and in one particular genetic miasm, *Tuberculinum*. I will describe what these are later on when I illustrate my own treatment.

The other major piece that still surprises me today is that as I began to let go, Jordan was able to surrender more to his own process. I now know that on that first day in Patty's office was the first advent in my quest to "let go." I had never trusted anyone else when it came to my own or my family's well-being and it was an intrinsic part of what I needed to do. In essence, Jordan was doing an awesome job of mirroring my unresolved emotional issues back to me as children are most often designed to do.

I was effectively hanging on to buckets of grief, fear, anger and guilt sustained over a course of a lifetime. His withheld stool was a physical representation of the "shit" I had not yet worked through.

Relinquish, acquiesce and yield were not terms I had ever grown familiar with. I had no real clue what they meant or how to embody them into my exhausted psyche. Out of fear, I had overcompensated in my efforts to avoid dealing with the grief which drove me to impose anger, blame and guilt to muscle my way through my whole life. My lopsided soul was like an enfeebled one-legged crab. I came to the conclusion that I had some serious work to do on myself if I was going to effectively help Jordan move through his issues.

CHAPTER 9

TREATING MOM

A s I witnessed Jordan's huge shifts, I could see the potential for my own healing. Intrinsically, I knew I was sitting on a number of time bombs given the unresolved emotional issues that I still carried from childhood. I was plagued with heavy grief and anger sustained from my mother's suicide when I was only eight years old and my father's early death from a heart attack when I was seventeen.

Beyond those events in my immediate family was the early death of my mother's sister who contracted a mysterious cancer that developed as a lump on her neck. Her brother, my uncle, was estranged for illicit behaviours including stealing money from his own mother. I have one surviving aunt who provides a link to the past.

My mother's father was deranged and he was committed to a mental institution when she was a child. I never knew him and hardly anyone ever spoke of him. I did track him down at one point while I was in university, however, both my aunts forbade me to see him and I respected their wishes.

I suspect that they must have sustained certain abuses for them to be so adamant. I modeled their retention of unspoken plights.

All in all, the obvious disease patterns that plagued my ancestral line were enough to make me shudder. At the time I decided to embark on treatment, I was not suffering with any particular rash of symptoms; however, I realized later, I was incurring enough danger signs and signals to indicate that I was on the verge of becoming a very sick woman.

Over time, the grief and anger from childhood events had begun to take their toll. I was overcome with a heaviness of both body and spirit. I gained a great deal of weight as I felt myself spiralling down with the feelings of abandonment. By my late 20s, I was 40 pounds overweight, very numb, and working for the government in a window-less eight-by-ten-foot cubicle. One day, I looked around and wondered, "How had I arrived here?" This was a place where my colleagues counted the months, weeks and hours until retirement. In essence, this is where my spirit had come to die.

As a child, I had occasionally woken up in the middle of the night with whole poems written in my head. I would glide out of bed to my desk to write them down before returning to sleep. I sang incessantly and used my own voice as a form of emotional therapy. I would find the most heart wrenching tunes and sing them with as much passion as I could muster, often collapsing in tears by the end. Patsy Cline is still one of my favourite crooners from that personal epoch!

I could play piano by ear and would spend countless hours at friends' houses playing the same tunes over and over again, until I'd worked out the melody. I also loved to draw and paint, but neither my education nor home-life were conducive to fostering creativity. Both were a void. So I began to undervalue these facets of my character and gradually let go of the things I loved to do. I was encouraged by others to just get through school and get a job working as a white-collar worker. This is what my parents had done and this should be enough for me.

By my late 20s, my poetic muse, my creative side, had been dormant for years. I made a smart and reasoned decision to marry a man who would be a dependable husband and responsible father. I was effectively numb to my feelings, so I based most of my decisions on cerebral calculations. He was a kind and loving white-collar worker and a good match for me!

By the time I embarked on treatment, I didn't have a host of firm symptoms that would seemingly qualify me for any medical treatment, but that doesn't mean that I didn't have a smattering of "energetic disturbances." By the time I faced the possibility of Heilkunst treatment, I was already calculating what kind of work I would have to do if I had to reverse something more significant like a tumour or heart disease later on.

I was not remotely aware of the cost incurred from suppressing my creativity. I just deemed my childhood ambitions to write, sing and paint to be fancies from another time. They couldn't possibly be viable beyond the category of "hobbies." It often felt as if that side of me had been fostered by another person and she had expired due to lack of interest. Besides, there were few "artistic types" in my biological family. There were many farmers, government employees and a couple of furniture salespersons so I guessed this was acceptable employment.

I was aware, though, that I had become very numb and very superficial in my daily functioning. I would get up in the morning, put on the black, brown or grey business suit, get my son to his sitter, and go to work for the required 7.5 hours per day. Nothing had much meaning or depth for me. I tried to ignore how exhausted I was all of the time. I would allow myself to lie in bed one day a month, read two or three magazines cover to cover, watch talk shows and sleep.

I collected recipes like crazy and I would tout that I prepared a different dish every night of the year. My husband used to joke that he would say "hello" and "goodbye" to a particular meal in the same breath, as he would never have the opportunity to sample it again.

I loved Victorian movies, like Pride and Prejudice, where the heroine suffered with her own inner truth to the point where she was about to lose everything, including "the guy," because she couldn't bring herself to bridge others' expectations of her. The abject misery in her life and mine was profound.

My friends would tease me about how clean my house was. If a chair or picture frame were a millimetre off kilter, I would get off the couch to straighten it. I would pluck a wilting leaf off a plant, never allowing it to completely die for fear I might expire in the process. My laundry never over-flowed and my bed linen was always changed once a week. You could have eaten off my floors!

I also had a habit that I could never drive the same route I had taken on the way to anywhere. An indescribable compulsiveness would always force me to find an alternate route home. This drove my husband crazy. He preferred routine and my idiosyncrasies were a source of bewilderment I'm sure. My home and my life were fastidious orchestrations of antiseptic madness.

So one frost-kissed October morning, I decided to take one drop from the low potency of the four emotional remedies for grief, anger, fear and guilt. I had made an appointment with Patty Smith, but that wasn't for another week and my confidence for prescribing acute self-limiting first-aid issues was getting to be old hat!

With my very first drop I unleashed what felt like a black ooze rising up the back of my legs, ascending further up my back and over my head like the cape of a cobra. I felt this profound shroud envelope me in every sense. My vision became tunnelled, I was not able to start or complete sentences as my thoughts were so fleeting and then they would just trail off. My mental acuity so deserted me that I could not drive the car or even speak on the phone. I fed the kids "picnic style" on the kitchen floor for three days as standing upright for any amount of time was too challenging. I was completely nauseated and beyond furious.

I felt as if a malevolent monster had been unleashed within and it swam like murky ooze between my bones and my skin. I was seething with an animosity so pure I felt almost murderous. Who had dared to unleash these dormant sceptres from within? I was getting my first taste of what Jordan might have been experiencing during his healing reactions. To say the least, I felt very anxious about being encased in black muck and mire and I went on a mission of blame.

I had obviously been storing energetic bucketfuls of all of these combined emotions and by taking the remedy, I had unwittingly invited them all to come out of their closets for a sardonic dance! I was immersed in my first "homeopathic healing reaction" and I was aggravated by a grief so tangible it was like an entity all its own, and its presence made me feel so vulnerable that I snapped caustically at anyone who dared come into my circle of influence. I was afraid beyond belief as I had always controlled these emotions and now they were obviously having their way with me and there wasn't a damn thing I could do about it. I felt so badly for every thought and subsequent word uttered that I just retreated into a numb funk to avoid any further confrontations. I didn't have the mental capacity to defend myself anyway and I certainly wasn't fit to live with. I wanted to escape the prison of "me" more than anyone!

I was also nursing my 10-month-old baby girl, Adie, at the time and I wondered how this seemingly mucky sludge in my veins was affecting her. She seemed to nurse normally and she didn't respond differently even though I was sure she must taste the vile bitterness I was feeling and I waited for her to react with some kind of "colic" at the very least.

Unlike allopathic drugs, although the combination remedy would have leeched through my breast milk, there are no side effects or risk of harming a baby who is still nursing. Fetuses' in-utero can even be safely treated with homeopathic remedies. In fact, my daughter Adie would have benefited from the low potencies I was taking. Like Jordan, she would be carrying a significant amount of my baggage anyway and the emotional remedies would just help her to clear these issues for herself.

During that time, I'm sure my husband thought that I was now completely unhinged and it was probably a good time to call "Shady Acres." For days, it seemed I clung to the precipice of my sanity. I couldn't believe that this healing reaction was all from one single drop of the remedy in one glass of water!

When I accusingly consulted my stepmother about the practices she obviously championed, she recommended that I further dilute the wee potion by pouring the remainder of the glass into another two glasses of water and sipping it only once or twice a day. She also remarked, "Wow, you certainly are sensitive!" I angrily replied, "I have always been that way and it seems like a heck of an oversight that everyone just recognizes this now!" She added, "Well, better out than in!" God, how I learned to hate that statement spouted regularly by her and Patty.

The truth is that I have rarely met other individuals who are as sensitive to the remedies as I was. After a week of continuously taking one or two sips of the diluted remedies, my head started to clear somewhat. Within two more days, I noticed some further improvements in my state of mind. It is so difficult to quantify, but I was thinking in ways that I had not thought in years. Formerly, if I read a three-frame comic strip, I was not able to remember the context of the first frame by the time I reached the third.

My thought patterns were becoming much clearer, and I felt less encumbered both physically and emotionally; lighter so to speak. One day while driving to work, I noticed the rich reds and golds of the fall leaves etched against the robin's egg blue sky. Colour started to have a profound impact on me and I began to crave more vibrant displays of nature.

At my initial consultation with Patty, I told her about my experience and she also seemed very excited that I had had such a profound healing reaction. I had wanted some sympathy for all that I had endured over the last two weeks and it seemed it was not forthcoming. I didn't get it. I had wallowed so long and so well in the pit of my emotional tomb that I was not keen to hear that it was time to let go. What would be left of me if I allowed all that defined me to slip away? The terror of letting go was so primal that it was beyond my comprehension. I could clearly see, now, what Jordan was expressing during his healing reactions. I too wanted to cause someone or something physical harm. I wondered if he also felt the need to hang on to everything that had authenticated his existence up until recently.

I never thought in this lifetime that I would take an opportunity to discharge the bucketfuls of stored anger, grief, fear and guilt from my core. Wow, what would that even look like? Would there really be anything left of me other than a vacuous shell? Everything I thought, everything I did was based on trying to keep it all stuffed down in the marrow of my bones. Could I sustain the charge if a meltdown to my core occurred? Surely the more noble organs would also opt to go!

On the flip side, however, what would my life look like if I were to remain encumbered with all of those negative emotions? What illnesses could potentially manifest from suppressing so much for so long? Was I prepared to continue to be defined by the pain and angst?

I remember that at that moment, I harnessed some inkling of strength that I had used to survive the deaths of my beloved parents. I was going to have to let go of my tightly woven neat little world and swim once more through the darkness of the void. I decided that not knowing the outcome was of less risk than allowing me to fully embrace disease. I began my own journey into the world of Heilkunst and homeopathy.

CHAPTER 10

THE JOURNEY BEGINS

I left Patty's office on October 30, 1998 with a commitment to my own healing and two more dropper bottles. I was instructed to write down my chief complaints and also a full timeline of all the emotional and physical traumas that had ever occurred to me over my lifetime. We would use this tool to map out my treatment. I had been to see therapists many times during my life, but I had never sat down and encapsulated the whole mess of afflictions in one exercise before.

I had been the type of person who could remember vividly back into my childhood, including the taste of the paint on the corners of my crib. I still had memories of what it was like to be a baby, standing in my crib and looking at the lamb wallpaper, my white dresser and the little blue lamb lamp, the curtains pulled and having just awoken from an afternoon nap. This is by no means a requirement for effective Heilkunst treatment as even those individuals who have been adopted are all effectively treated; however, I have had distinct glimpses similar to this one throughout my childhood. Through disease, I had almost entirely lost this awareness.

So I sat down one evening and wrote out my present chief complaints. I included the hypoglycemia that plagued me. Often my blood sugar would dip so low that I would break into a cold sweat, feeling panicky and faint. I also documented the chronic fatigue and muscle aches. Every time a low-pressure system moved in, I was in bed with a headache that felt as if there were vice grips on my temples. I had shingles on my right shoulder, which further manifested as a patch of rashy blisters and the mirror image of the same on the upper right side of my chest. The nerves in my right arm were always numb and tingling and I would often drop things, as I could not fully sense when I had picked them up or not. I always had canker sores inside my bottom lip and psoriasis on the perimeter of my scalp. The doctor had labeled me with premenstrual syndrome and dysmenorrhea in my early 20s.

Once, when I was pregnant with Jordan, I was at the grocery store. I remember finding myself in one of the aisles completely lost. I had no idea how I had arrived or why I was there. I just began to weep and thankfully my husband found me in amongst the canned goods and took me home. Sadly, this type of situation was happening more frequently in my life. I would break down for seemingly no reason and cry for hours, hot tears burning my cheeks and swelling my eyelids for days afterwards.

The flip side of that was the way I blamed absolutely everyone and everything for every little inconvenience that plagued me. This litany of events riddled my life and fed my irritability and rage. There was little or no congruency between my actions and my state of mind.

If we were going away for the weekend, I secretly desired to be home alone. Because of my perceived powerlessness, I would vomit at the curb on the way to my in-laws. I always felt trapped, like an innocent, wrongly jailed and constantly victimized by the jailers. I had no clue what freedom would look like. And although I felt incarcerated in my present circumstances, I did not possess the ego structure to figure out what I truly wanted. So I imagined that I was just being dragged from one place to another. At least I could blame the other party for my misery when I got there. I hated my circumstances. I took no responsibility for myself and allowed myself to be "done to." I was the eternal victim.

I remember crying out for help on a number of occasions. One day when I was 18, I was sitting on the stairs in a house I was living in while at university. My period was so heavy, I was gushing with blood and clots so voluminous, that I worried I was bleeding to death. I called my doctor who told me he had other more significant issues to face and that I should just go and lie down.

While making scrambled eggs the next morning, I fainted on the kitchen floor and was taken to hospital, where I was diagnosed with dysmenorrhoea. However, knowing that I had a label did not change anything. I suffered for years pent up at home during that time of the month, waiting for the heavy bleeding to taper off enough that I could go about "living."

Once, when the abdominal pains were severe, I carted myself off to the hospital. A scope was inserted into my navel and all they found was an inflamed bowel. I had introduced myself to the spicy eclectic foods of the big city on my way to falling in love with the spicy nature of its ethnic people. My background was so bland "white bread" that I had worked hard to erase all residues of my suburban middle class upbringing.

I danced with a variety of drugs that coloured my bland existence. I used LSD, mushrooms and cocaine when I could afford them. I never went to sleep without smoking hashish before bed for over a year. I particularly enjoyed the clean, euphoric feeling from cocaine, which I would have considered a permanent vice had I had the money to support it.

I had suffered chronic bladder, kidney and yeast infections since my teen years. Every month after my period, the corrosive yeast would invade undergarments and cause so much itchiness that I would want to tear at myself with nails for relief. Two days later, the burning pain in my urethra would begin where urinating would become so painful, I would hold the walls of bathroom stalls and suppress screams. Often when I urinated, blood would fill the toilet bowl. This went on month after month for years. Occasionally, it would move into my kidneys and I would end up at the doctor's office with another prescription for Erythromycin™.

I suffered with bouts of chronic sinus infections that would last weeks during the winter months. Once when I was pregnant with Jordan, I had one so bad that

I had the urge to bang my head against the doorframe just to see if that would help ease the unbearable pressure in my head. Sleeping was next to impossible as I thought my head was going to explode. I was often up snorting nasal decongestants during the night in an effort to clear my nasal passages enough to sleep for a couple more hours.

My emotional timeline included giving birth to both of my children, my conversion to Judaism to marry my husband and the resultant feelings of loss of identity, wisdom teeth extractions, other minor surgeries, constant exposure to chlorine as a competitive swimmer, the experimental drug use in university, and the death of my 43-year-old father of a sudden heart attack in 1981 when I was 17. And then we moved back further in time to my Dad's marriage to my stepmother in 1972 and then in 1971, when I was seven, I had incurred the most devastating trauma of my life, the suicide of my biological mother. I loved her with incredible and pure abandon. I was so mystified by the act as I also knew how much she loved me. I asked myself sometimes hourly for years, "How could she just up and leave me here all alone?"

Throughout my treatment I was continuously amazed at how much of my emotional baggage was profoundly anchored here. I waded through the buckets of grief and anger to get at the bottom of this very grimy inner swamp. I knew the primal shadow resided in its depths.

The last two events to clear on my timeline were my vaccination shocks and my own birth trauma. My mom's blood type was "Rh negative" and there may have been complications that I am not aware of, so we treated it as if I had had a blood transfusion since no one surviving in my family could tell me. A relative of mine was unsure, but she remembered that either my sister or I had received one.

Like Jordan, each event on my timeline would be treated sequentially using the homeopathic remedies at each follow-up appointment, at approximately four-week intervals. My onion was going to be effectively peeled one layer at a time!

This approach to treatment has been applied effectively for more than ten years by Patty Smith and Rudolf Verspoor in their Clinic. As mentioned earlier, their particular therapeutic application using homeopathic remedies was further developed and grounded on their collaborative research with Steven Decker.

Steven and Rudi had worked together to write a number of books on the subject including *The Dynamic Legacy: From Homeopathy to Heilkunst*, which describes the principles and philosophy of this medical system. At present, it is available as a vast electronic library that encompasses a broad range of treatment jurisdictions based on this sound research. Rudi has often said that this principled system for cure was always just sitting there waiting for anyone to see it; however, we may not have been ready until now.

CHAPTER 11

THE TIMELINE APPROACH

Individuals store, energetically, every emotional and physical trauma that they have ever incurred. If you've had a car accident, for example, ten years later, you may develop a chronic soreness in your neck. You can see your chiropractor to try to manage the pain or get an anti-inflammatory from your doctor to suppress it, but the root of the issue has not been addressed, and so you may find that it recurs or starts to spawn other symptoms like headaches. Clinically, Heilkunst has proven that by addressing the timeline event, the root is annihilated and the symptoms no longer have anywhere to anchor.

This is very interesting to witness and I will recall a story that I hope illustrates this phenomena well:

We were vacationing in New Brunswick the summer that Jordan turned four years old. One night my husband and I heard a very loud cry from the bedroom Jordan was sleeping in. When we went to him, we discovered that he had fallen out of bed onto the floor. Naturally, Jordan was very upset, but my husband crawled into bed with him and soon both of them fell back to sleep. The next morning, and each day after that, Jordan asked that I be careful putting his shirt over his head as he said his neck hurt. He continued to play with his cousins, ride roller coasters and swing a putter like a pro without any complaint. Admittedly, he spent a great deal of time with family and I did not notice that something was really wrong until we were driving back to Ottawa.

On the way home, we stopped at a hotel and I was playing catch with him. To my horror, I noticed that one of his arms was dangling lower than the other. Upon our arrival in Ottawa the next day, we went straight to the clinic where an x-ray revealed that Jordan's collarbone was broken cleanly through. I felt devastated. Jordan's arm was immobilized in a sling and I started treating him with the appropriate remedies once we arrived home.

Eighteen months later, during the course of Jordan's treatment, he woke up one morning with a very stiff neck and crying in pain. When I asked him where it hurt, he showed me and further explained that it felt exactly like it did when he fell out of the bed in New Brunswick. I called Patty right away, as I did not recall treating this event on his timeline. Patty let me know that we had not recorded this event on his timeline and it quickly became clear to me that I had probably overlooked it. I must have blocked it from my memory due to the guilt I harboured over my lack of awareness during his plight.

We "backed up" an event in Jordan's timeline to treat the one that had come up for our viewing pleasure, Jordan's "neck pain" resolved itself in less than 24 hours and we were able to continue onto the next event.

The interesting thing to me was how Jordan intuitively knew what key phrase to use in order to spark my memory around his sore neck. If he had not used precisely those words, it was very likely that I might never have registered the true nature of his complaint and thereby missed the potential for closure on this incident. I was starting to trust in some of the "occurrences" that began to emerge over the course of our treatment.

The dropper bottles that accompanied me home after my initial consultation with Patty were very accurately prescribed. The first one was for a patient who, under stress, becomes progressively more detached from family and community.

There can be marked irritability, depression and indifference, and any demand by the family is viewed as a further burden and might be met with resignation or anger. You might even see examples of these very stressed out parents at the shopping mall shrieking at their children and unable to control their temper. Patty gave me the classic remedy prescribed for care-worn and overwhelmed housewives who crave nothing more than to be alone. This described my state of mind to a tee.

Sepia is the remedy derived from the ink sac of the cuttlefish. Dr. Douglas Gibson[6] suggests that the ink sac of the cephalopod is the same as the gall bladder in vertebrates. Bile, gall and biliousness are synonymous with black depression in the human. Depression is a prominent feature of the *Sepia* state. Of all the cephalopods, cuttlefish have the largest supply of ink for their size and are the most ready to use it! So, based on the law of similars, when treated with the remedy *Sepia*, it would help address my anger, black depression and my deposits of verbal rage when seemingly attacked.

When my kids were very young, I had felt very much like a guitar string that was wound too tightly. I always felt that I had never had the required love and nurturing needed during my own childhood in order to effectively deal with the stresses of mothering two children of my own and running a household in addition to working full-time. I was finding it increasingly challenging to remain at any task long-term, as I always arrived at a state of exhaustion and utter desolation in almost everything that I undertook. I felt stuck in childhood patterns without the tools to move forward. While others would evolve into the next stage of their lives, I wanted to go back and fill the voids with the missed nurturing.

I attributed this to my unresolved issues around abandonment by my mother. In my mind, everything had a short lifespan and if there was effectively nothing feeding me, I was out of there. From her death to the present day, I had been on a mission to find sources of replacement for the love I craved. As a result I made inexhaustible demands on my husband. The only difference between the dysfunction in my family and his were that I was dealing solely with ghosts. He was still dealing, or rather, not dealing with moving targets.

I felt that there was never enough of me to go around and it always seemed someone or something always wanted more from me than I was able to effectively give. So, it was no surprise to me that I found it stifling to try to parent from a vacuum where there did not appear to be any fuel forthcoming for my impoverished spirit. Certainly, I looked for this void to be filled within my marriage, and again, there was no surprise to realize that the capacity to fill my depleted cavity did not lie with my husband either. While we both blamed the state we found ourselves in on the isolation we felt from any familial support, we also knew that a primary connection was also missing between us. We would honour our intimacy once every month or so as a duty to our marriage. We entered the realm of psychological therapy over the next year to try to address the root of our issues. These things had plagued our marriage from very early on.

The second remedy was for my constitution. This is a term used to describe one's predisposition or character typology. Understanding these archetypal personalities enables one to understand those behaviours and emotional tendencies that influence each of them. Each one of the six "genotypes" will face different internal conflicts and spiritual issues and knowing the characteristics of your own constitution can provide you with insights concerning how you behave within and without throughout your life.

The medicinal reason for taking the constitutional remedy is to help balance the Sustentive power. If an individual sleeps with the window open throughout winter, craves chips every day, and talks to her mother four times a day at the age of 38, you may find that these eccentricities are more balanced after a dose of the person's constitutional remedy.

People love to study this facet of homeopathy as it can be likened to the astrological sun signs where we can derive a clear picture of certain typologies based on the formation of the stars in the galaxy at the time you were born. Some people are also familiar with the Four Temperaments or Humours first coined by Empedocles of Akragas (432 BC). He was a Greek philosopher who was a subscriber to the Pythagorean School of natural philosophers and he postulated that all substances were made up of air, earth, fire, and water combined in different proportions later adopted by Hippocrates whose medical methodology and ethics are still practised today. The four Temperaments are Sanguine, Phlegmatic, Choleric and Melancholic and also refer to personality characteristics deduced from the Etheric body or our interrelationship with nature.

CHAPTER 12

WHAT'S A CONSTITUTION?

When Jordan and I both began Heilkunst treatment, we were asked a series of questions to determine our homeopathic constitution. "Are you generally hot or cold? Do you sleep with the covers on or do you kick them off during the night? Do you prefer salty, spicy or sweet foods? Are you an introverted sort or extroverted?" are examples.

This line of questioning can lead to the determination of a patient's "constitutional type." Administering a "constitutional" remedy can help even out those extreme elements in our personality and lend support during healing reactions.

For example, the *Phosphorous* constitution loves salt. If I were eating ten bags of chips per day, taking the *Phosphorous* remedy could annihilate this out-of-whack craving and help restore my balance.

A healing reaction is defined as the bi-product of our Life Force acting to restore balance against disease. When a remedy is given, your body acts like a slingshot preparing to fire a rock. The sling is pulled back, stretched to its limits and then released. If we imagine the disease flying like a rock out of the body of the sling, the elastic band then comes back to a place of rest. The body comes back to a place of rest too, but slightly different than before. It then has the job of re-calibrating itself on all levels in order to adjust without the prior disease in its midst. This re-calibration happens on all levels of your being – the mental, physical, emotional and spiritual. The healing reaction is the re-calibration of your system. It is also known as the "counter-action."

By learning to live without the prior disease, you can obtain a new kind of freedom. In addition to a lessening of symptoms, perceptible feelings of being less encumbered, clearer in thinking and an ability to sustain stresses more easily are some of the benefits I've witnessed first hand.

A constitutional genotype is easily identified when you are in a state of health and balance. Sometimes, these archetypal characteristics are not easily discernible if there are layers of grief, anger or other fundamentals of disease cloaking these true states of being. And although, in some cases the genotype is not easily discernible, stripping off layers of trauma will usually reveal it before too long.

The clinical research indicates that patients do feel more balanced and are able to sustain the charge of their healing reactions more easily. However, it is sort of like providing the icing on the proverbial cake of disease. It makes the dry cake part much more palatable. The founder of this system of medicine, Dr. Samuel Hahnemann stated in his *Organon of the Medical Art* that, "The Physician's highest and *only* calling is to make the sick healthy, to cure, as it is called."[7]

So while treating someone's constitution can be beneficial, all physicians have one sole responsibility and that is to cure disease and support the healing process. When guided by principles, this is very cut and dried. The sole purpose of medicine is to destroy the disease(s) in patients, which entails provoking the healing reaction on the part of the patient's Life Force. That's it, that's all!

The treatment of the constitution really falls under "supporting the healing process." This has a powerful jurisdiction of its own which falls more in the realm of "sustaining health" using the law of opposites. As per Verspoor and Decker, the use of this particular law of nature is considered to be valid in two ways: to add what is lacking or subtract what is in excess. So if someone is Vitamin C deficient, you give them more Vitamin C. If someone is developing shin splints from running on pavement, suggest a bit of rest and a softer, grassier plain. You can also use the remedies effectively in an area of treatment where there is an absence of disease. The constitution is one of these areas.

Now, let's take a look at the characteristics of the various constitutions. The six genotypes can be split into two quadrants: one being the upper spiritual pole, or those constitutions that derive their characteristics from the cosmos, and the other being the lower spiritual pole or those constitutions that derive their characteristics from the earth pole.

In the upper pole there is *Silicea, Phosphorous* and *Lycopodium* and in the lower pole, *Pulsatilla, Calcarea carb* and *Sulphur*. (Don't worry about the German words associated with the constitutions closest to the bottom of the diagram. They are terms that are difficult to translate and so we learn to intuit the meanings of them over three years of study.) It may be easier if you visualize them like this:

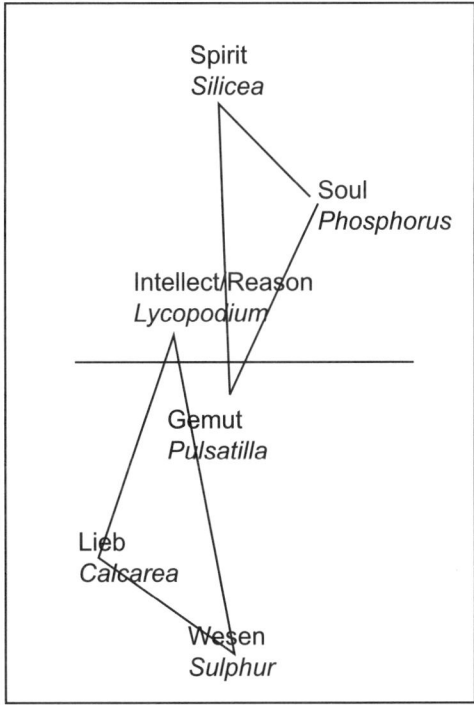

Source: Verspoor and Decker; Dynamic Legacy: From Homeopathy to Heilkunst [8]

The centre line may leave you asking questions about *Lycopodium* and *Pulsatilla* regarding which triad they truly belong to. This is a great question, as the intellect often desires to compartmentalize or carve things up only one way. There are in fact two ways to conceptualize *Pulsatilla* and *Lycopodium*. They are the only two constitutions that are derived from plants whereas all of the others are derived from the mineral kingdom. *Pulsatilla nigricans* is a fragile wind-flower and *Lycopodium clavatum* is also known as club moss. And the latter is not always sure whether it is a moss or fern. While the mineral types are fairly solid and immovable in their characteristics, changeability is indicative of both *Pulsatilla* and *Lycopodium* given that a plant is required to sustain environmental stresses in order to survive. Therefore, while *Pulsatilla* is considered in the upper triad, they are also quite emotional and earthy. And, although *Lycopodium* is truly considered part of the earth triad, they are intellectually bent and often hyper-conscientious which is more indicative of characteristics derived from the upper pole. We will look at each of these in detail in the next chapter.

There are six other constitutional types or "states" that we define as phenotypes which result from trauma, strains and stresses on the healthy genotype. I mentioned earlier how I was prescribed *Sepia* at one of my first consultations with Patty, and given the stresses and strains of mothering under arduous conditions with little or no reprieve and the prevailing feelings that I was "not enough" given my traumatic past, I had a tendency to dance into this state on and off depending on circumstances.

A phenotype can appear just like a genotype except "with a twist of lime!" Rudolf Verspoor writes, "They appear in individuals who have been subjected to a series of traumas, such as death in the family, abuse or a divorce or to the suppression of their natural creative (sexual) energy."[9]

Under such stress, the constitutional state can shift into a secondary one, which we call the phenotype. In essence, when stresses are sustained by the primary constitution against the backdrop of the chronic miasms and false beliefs, the original state of health cannot maintain its solidarity. In answer, the secondary phenotype is created as a defence and the state of health shifts in response to the presence of disease.

These secondary remedies represent the result of the suppression or repression of the natural flow of generative energy in a state of health, either at the psychic level or the physical level.

This adds further evidence to the work of Dr. Wilhelm Reich in the first part of this century on the development of Freud's distinction between psychoneurosis and actual (stasis) neurosis. "Based on our understanding of the remedies (through the materia medica) and of the concepts of Reich's psychoneurosis (blockage of energy stemming from internal prohibitions, termed repression) and stasis neurosis (blockage of energy from the suppressive impingement of the environment), we can divide the six remedies into two groups."[10]

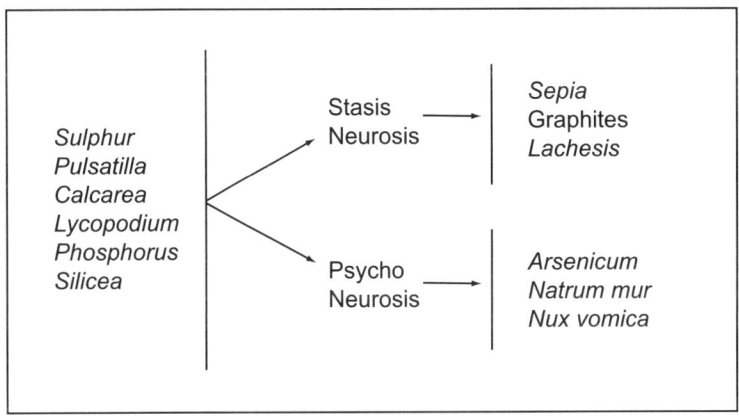

Source: Verspoor and Decker; Dynamic Legacy: From Homeopathy to Heilkunst [11]

It may be important to note that this is a living system of medicine and changes are bound to occur as further research illumines initial hypotheses. "*Graphites*" has been replaced by *Staphysagria* (remedy for anger) on the chart above. The other thing to remember is that genotypes define your characteristics when you are in a state of Health. Dr. Douglas Gibson, Philip M. Bailey, Rajan Sankaran and Catherine Coulter have all written great books illustrating the characteristics of the constitutions; however, you should keep in mind that their research is primarily based on patients who are not necessarily healthy, and their descriptions contain a mix of healthy characteristics along with elements of disease or imbalance. Also, the classical dogma makes no distinction between health and disease, no acknowledgement of a typology of six healthy constitutions, so all remedies (thousands of them!) are wrongly considered "constitutions." So you will have to do some detective work to discern the healthy characteristics from the unhealthy ones. For example, according to Dr. Douglas Gibson the chief characteristics of a *Silicea* patient are:

"extreme inertia, lack of response, lack of fire and very poor resistance. The grain of sand is content to drift, subside and settle motionless on the surface of the desert or on the seabed, away beneath the waves of bother and strife. The *Silicea* patient just wants to sit around or lie down in apparent unconcern. But if provoked he may blow up over trifles and become violent, even as the sand of the desert, if stirred up, may become a whirl of violence and destructiveness."[12]

Although I love reading Dr. Gibson's *Studies of Homeopathic Remedies*, as he does an awesome job of connecting us to their natural sources, I often feel a lack of resonance as I know many healthy *Siliceas* who do not elicit characteristics remotely close to these. In fact, most of what is cited in accounts about constitutions by other authors is also quite skewed for the same reason.

My father was a dependable, warm and kind *Silicea* and my first husband was very much like him, and my son, Jordan, is the most outgoing and emotionally connected one I know. I can't remotely imagine describing anyone of them this way. I work and study with *Siliceas* who have been Heilkunst treated and I have even adopted another as part of my family and so I am always a little taken aback when I unearth references like this.

I am hoping that as the system of homeopathy and Heilkunst evolves, that we will be able to give birth to a healthier reference so that a clearer, more accurate picture of each genotype and phenotype can be accessed by this blossoming community.

CHAPTER 13

WHICH CONSTITUTION ARE YOU?

In the mid-1990s, Daniel Goleman, a Harvard psychology PhD wrote, *Emotional Intelligence: Why It Can Matter More Than IQ for Character, Health and Lifelong Achievement.*[13] In his best-seller, he cites that it is no longer true that industry and academic institution only value a person's IQ. He cites that "emotional intelligence, or EQ, gives you a competitive edge." While that may be true, the constitutional typology also values the differences between EQ intelligence and IQ intelligence. While EQs will derive their energy from being with other people, IQ's will prefer solitude to recharge their weary batteries. As you go through the descriptions of each genotype, you will quickly discern the difference between them.

A *Silicea* is closest to the Spirit or "*Geist*" pole and we can often identify them physically as the tall, lean, refined and elegant creature they are as they seem to stretch themselves closer to the cosmos even on a physical level. They are IQ types and derive energy from being alone. They are often noted for their intellectual prowess, logic and sense of righteousness and justice. They can be quite reserved and cool emotionally and they often have to stretch themselves to relate to their feelings and risk allowing others into their inner world.

They are often quite delicate and often have to be mindful of their regimen as it is best if they get adequate sleep and food at regular intervals. They are often mentally preoccupied and they will be known to forget to eat which can weaken them considerably. They are known to wear warmer clothes than the average and both adults and children often need to be reminded that, "the seasons have changed, snow hasn't fallen for two weeks, so put away the winter galoshes!"

Silicea is silicon dioxide, which occurs in nature as quartz, flint sandstone and many other substances. It is important to note that this element is often used in industry due to its non-reactivity and resistance to oxidation.

A *Silicea* child needs time alone and a loud, overbearing or critical style of parenting can seriously compromise their quality of life and will often produce a phenotype in response. They also need to be gently encouraged to put down their book until later and go outside to play as nature helps to ground them.

Siliceas are usually a pleasure to parent as they are sensitive and aware of boundaries well before overt discipline is required. However, they struggle with change and their risk taking is usually kept to a minimum, so they most likely will be your last child to leave home. You may want to delay turning their bedroom into a solarium until you are sure they are really gone!

Phosphorous is also close to the spirit pole and they are considered the soul of all constitutional genotypes, the fundamental quality of soul being expression and expressivity of being. They are EQ types and you usually know that you are in the presence of one when you are mesmerized by their sparkling eyes and bubbly personality. They can also be emotionally cool as they can live very much in the moment and when you leave the room, you are truly forgotten which can be a bit disconcerting to some. They are fun to be with; however, if you find you feel uncomfortable in their presence, it is often due to their lack of boundaries. They are known to stir up people's emotions unnecessarily or necessarily depending on how you look at it. They are bright, popular and magnetic and we often love to be with them if we suffer from ennui in our own lives. They usually possess inherent psychic abilities and their intuition can be quite remarkable. *Phosphorous* can often get frustrated with how society does not generally value their strengths as they are often perceived as flighty or unable to persevere when tasks become routine or mundane. They thrive in a changeable environment which is not usually an acceptable standard for IQ types.

Phosphorous is usually very attractive physically and energetically and you can often spot them matchmaking with a twinkle in their eye. They make great travel agents, talent scouts, and writers of children's books as their playful imagination remains keen throughout their lives.

Phosphorous is an element essential to life, whether animal or vegetable. Its presence, for instance, is necessary for the transfer of energy within plant cells through chemical reactions. The first substance, newly absorbed from the atmosphere that has been shown to be present in a plant also includes phosphorous.

The physical properties of phosphorous are noteworthy. By reason of its combustibility in air at normal temperatures, it has to be stored under water or in alcohol. When exposed to the air it oxidizes and rises into the atmosphere. Phosphorous is the green iridescence seen on the surface of the ocean and I love how these types are so much about light without an identifiable source of heat. Their boundless energy just seems to be derived from within. They will usually have a great love for the sun, a fear of thunder and things that go bump in the night so your *Phosphorous* child may spend more time in your bed than their siblings of different constitutions.

Pulsatillas live by their gut instinct or intuition. To describe what most characterizes them, we use the German word Gemüt, for which there is no direct translation into English. Steven Decker translated it as "emotional mind" in Hahnemann's sixth edition of *The Organon of the Medical Art*, edited by Wenda Brewster O'Reilly.

Pulsatillas are warm, earthy and often very maternal. Their connection to family is quite profound and they are usually surrounded by those they love since they prefer company over solitude. A *Pulsatilla* child will often absorb love and attention, but is not known to return it the same way a *Phosphorous* child does. Some *Pulsatillas* are prone to blush, to timidity and to imagined fears. However, I know many *Pulsatillas* who withstand many of life's changes and weather them very well without dissolving under pressure. By nature, they are very sensitive, but not as tenderhearted, sullen, discouraged, placid, yielding or craving attention as pictured in most Materia Medicas. At present, I have a *Pulsatilla* friend who calls quite regularly just to chat and talk about her latest reaction to a remedy. They like to be consoled and they can easily put into words how they are feeling, which are one of their favourite pastimes, and this makes them a pleasure to listen to!

Traditionally, they are often depicted as plump, cherubic types with changeable natures. They are also known for their chameleon-like abilities and they work well in environments where they can don a variety of personas. The risk to a *Pulsatilla* is losing themselves to other's expectations. *Pulsatilla* males also may have many challenges in this regard as society's expectations can be damaging to this sensitive, loving and gentle soul and we see many of them resorting to the protective armour intrinsic in a phenotype.

Pulsatilla Nigricans, the windflower, meadow anemone, or pasque flower can be strikingly beautiful and their yellowish gold or purplish blooms often grow in clumps in chalky soil primarily in England and Europe. Gibson cites that, "even the smell from the bruised leaves or broken flowers has been known to cause headache or fainting fits and to produce inflammation of the eyes. *Pulsatillas* are known to cleanse toxins quite heavily through their sinuses. Handling many blooms causes a form of eczema on the hands, and if the juice enters any cut or scratch a very serious sore may develop."[14]

Lycopodium Clavatum has the potential to operate in the realm of pure reason and intellect when unencumbered by disease. They are "cool" emotionally and very rational and pragmatic in their thinking. These types are orderly, conscientious, socially adept, adaptive and politically astute. They are very aware of hierarchies and they know how to work them to their advantage. *Lycopodium* people know how to dress well and you will find they are well groomed. They care very much about how they appear and they can be seen catching a glance at themselves in a mirror at the boss's swanky cocktail party. Social status is very important to these types and I have a *Pulsatilla* friend who blushes and apologizes for the size and obvious statement her beautiful home makes as she demurs, "It's not me who wants all this, but my *Lycopodium* husband!"

The *Lycopodium* individual is intellectually active, must be occupied as they find relief in action, movement and exercise, especially outdoors. *Lycopodium* loves soup to be hot when served, but will often suffer from gastric complaints and so will his family if they happen to walk by the bathroom after he has had a bowel movement!

These types cannot easily bear criticism, to be found at fault or opposed and they can become almost frantic if harassed through vexing or petty attacks. This is often the high priced Litigation Lawyer, the Member of Parliament or the very polished State Governor. We've all been surprised at the reaction of some politicians when confronted with an overt indiscretion. They will often lose their slick appearance and handle themselves in shockingly childish ways. Underneath the slick businessperson veneer, can be an insecure little boy or girl. They may have been raised with constant expectations around social or scholarly achievement which fuels their motivation to keep achieving this end so that they can finally feel accepted. Unfortunately, it can be a bit like the horse running after the carrot that is attached to his headgear. Finally, the variability in their personalities can be minimized when the *Lycopodium* defines their own ego structure independent of others' expectations.

I have witnessed *Lycopodium* individuals who, after doing two degrees at university, will claim that, "the law degree was for my father and the art history degree is for me." This is time consuming, but a healthier approach to the tides that pervade in these individuals.

As mentioned earlier, *Lycopodium* or wolf's claw is also known as club moss, lamb's tail, or fox tail which may give you an indication of its appearance. It lies somewhere between a moss and a fern which also illustrates its indeterminate classification as if it is of two minds. It grows abundantly on open mountain pastures in Europe and South Africa, throwing out long, prickly, straggly shoots that end in a forked tongue. *Lycopodium* can have a biting sarcasm and a proclivity for being pig-headed, and over conscientious.

The stems bear fruit filled with sporophylls that when shaken out will rain down a seemingly inert, odourless and tasteless yellow powder. I recently witnessed a memorable demonstration by Chemist Albert Schmidli, from Weleda

International, Switzerland who came to speak at a summer conference hosting Anthroposophical and Heilkunst Physicians. His purpose was to illustrate nature in her finest alchemic glory so that we homeopaths could remain mindful of how our remedies are derived and the corresponding transmuting effects they have on diseases in our patients.

Lycopodium spores contain about 50 per cent fixed oil, chiefly Lycopodiumoleic acid, also sugar, phytosterin, traces of alumia, phosphoric acid and silica. They are considered medicinally inert in the natural state. Mr. Schmidli opened a little bag full of the yellow powder and began to spoon the contents into his open mouth. He had a lit blowtorch at the ready and he proceeded to blow the contents of his mouth into the flame. For a moment, I thought I might be at a 1970s "KISS" concert as the flame ignited and exploded into a fireball that trailed high into the air and even down the laboratory table well across the floor. This was a real testament to the hidden powers of this extraordinary remedy and the hidden aspects of this character we know as *Lycopodium.*

Calcarea carbonica is represented by the Leib, or the body. Affectionately known as "*Calcs,*" these types are quite affable and easy going. They are very dependable and solid in their relationships. They make awesome parents as they are naturally very loving. Setting boundaries comes quite easily out of their tenacious, often stubborn side. Their children claim that, "once they've made up their mind, they are immovable!" Although, *Siliceas* can also exhibit stubbornness around ideas, *Calcs* will not want to be rushed into a decision or action. They gravitate towards routine and constancy provides them with a security necessary to their well-being. They don't mind repetitive jobs and they enjoy building systems that structure and govern how things are done. They love a systematic approach to everything!

Physically, they can tend towards being overweight as they are not as motivated to be active as other constitutions are. Dr. Gibson writes that, they, "principally mirror the general retardation deriving from disordered calcium metabolism."[15] The *Calc carb* subject is slow, dull, uninterested and timid, and shuns any form of mental effort … Fear is a marked feature. The *Calc carb* subject is full of fear – fear of people, fear of the dark, fear of being looked at, fear of solitude, a vague fear of "scarcely knows what," and "a growing fear of impending insanity."

Gibson goes even further to suggest that the sufferer of this state cannot stop thinking about his apprehension, and he is sure everyone is aware of his insecurity and is regarding him with suspicion. Again, it is very important to remember that this portrait is of an individual in a very unhealthy state. It is interesting to note that stress will increase for these types if their level of calcium is compromised so it is important to see whether this can be corrected through diet and exercise alone.

The source of this constitution is the soft, snowy-white calcareous substance in the middle layer of the oyster's shell, which is excreted by the mantle of the mollusk and is in fact a deposit of finely crystalline calcium carbonate.

It is interesting to notice the links between the constitution typology and the oyster's behaviour in its environment. Falling somewhere between a snail and a cuttlefish, it squats on the ocean floor with the two halves of its shell gaping widely, trapping food that happens to pass through by current. If the oyster should notice the slightest threat in its vicinity, it will invoke a muscular spasm to snap its shell closed with vice grip firmness.

Calcs tend to be clammy to the touch and quite often suffer with muscle spasms. Also their clam-like unresponsiveness is often just a mask that conceals agitation and anxiety within. As a parent of one of these individuals, I would be mindful of helping them define their stresses in order to provide a release. Their daily regimen would have to be monitored closely to ensure that their diet met their blood type and metabolic needs. They also require sufficient exercise and sleep to reduce any stress-induced toxicity. From my personal standpoint, *Calcarea carbonicas* are amazing people and I have had the pleasure of being invited into their warm and loving oyster shells. As someone who has sustained much trauma due to voids in nurturing and many changes in principal caregivers during my life, I know exactly why I've attracted these individuals as intimates.

Sulphur is derived from the Earth and defined by Verspoor as, "the pure instinct, the wise *Dynamis* in the organism. It is that entity which is the unchanging quintessence of something. It is not material, yet it is real. It permeates the whole of something and cannot be considered as separate from that something."[16]

Each one of us contains these "bodies" to a varying degree. In a healthy state, we should be influenced by all the constitutions, even though our predominant constitution will always remain constant.

Sulphurs are usually detected before they enter the room as their energy precedes them! They are passionate, "living for the moment" explorers who exhibit a fearless, open and earthy approach to life. They have big ideas and are often inventing the "machine" that is going to save humanity from endless toil. They have a black and white way of looking at the world and many will say that they are rather argumentative as they seem driven by their egos to confrontation. *Sulphurs* "think outside the box" and they are naturally self-educated, tactile learners who are unfortunately usually defined as Attention Deficit Hyper Disorder (ADHD) by allopathic doctors and now, even by teachers, who have begun to empower themselves as diagnosticians of this "so called" condition.

Unfortunately, our education system is not designed to tolerate these generous, inspired, reactive students who know that for them, "experience is the best teacher." These children need more time learning outside the classroom walls in connection with nature. The biggest challenge for a *Sulphur* child is to be told to sit at a desk and concentrate on seemingly meaningless equations on a piece of paper. I have, however, seen many of these children succeed in a Waldorf-based education system where they are encouraged to be in touch with nature and learn in a more feeling, tactile environment.

Although, individuals labelled with the condition ADHD can also have a great miasmic (genetic predisposition for disease) load, a lot can be accomplished by treating for their constitution alone. I have witnessed the eradication of these tendencies many times through Heilkunst treatment. Parents are stunned that their children are restored to a state of balance and emotional grace. If they are wise, they will also undergo treatment, as we know that it is often their baggage that has exacerbated the issues with the child. I speak from personal experience.

Sulphur is all about heat! They are quick-tempered, have passionate love-affairs and will tend to ignite over issues they care deeply about. These types think their own performances and possessions are of paramount worth and excellence and you may be in a position to hear about it. They make great trial lawyers, business coaches, interior designers, actors and inventors. They can have deeply held insecurities which can make them feel somewhat paranoid.

Sulphurs can also appear to be quite bright and even brilliant at times and then lapse into indolence or incoherence, if they are pushed to act on their ideas. It can seem almost impossible to get *Sulphur* to build some kind of structure or executable plan. They may feel that it is enough that they grace us with their creative smarts and then it is up to the rest of us to define the structure to carry out the plan.

A *Sulphur* woman who used to work in my office never washed her own dishes, participated in the annual yard clean-ups or shovelled the walkway which was a requirement of the cooperative environment in which we worked. She would tell us all how best to go about all the major projects, but her "Queenly" airs never allowed her to actually participate! When we jokingly brought it to her attention, she would act much like Teflon and let the remarks roll off her back. We all loved her and she taught me how to let go more around the rigid expectations with which I was raised.

Sulphur is a bright yellow rock, which burns to choking fumes, and has been used medicinally since early civilization. Homer wrote, "Bring me fire, that I may purify the house with sulphur."

Both *Phosphorous* and *Sulphur* are remedies which are associated with burning; both in a literal and physical sense. They clinically show up in symptoms of burning and heat in patients.

However, sulphur possesses opposite propensities to phosphorous, unlike the latter element which, when ignited by spontaneous combustion, disappears upwards in an ascending vapour. When Albert Schmidli, the Swiss Chemist, burned sulphur, there was a blue flame and its vapour re-condensed at normal surface temperature to form a yellow crystalline powder. This element and the constitution share an earthward tendency, a preoccupation with material things rather than art, a penchant for down-to-earth schemes as opposed to poetic fancy, and a predisposition for physical awareness rather than imaginings and extrasensory perceptiveness.

CHAPTER 14

CONSTITUTIONS AND LOVE

M ost people are very curious about which character typologies go best together if they are considering a mate. Of course it may be too late if you are already married to the wrong one! But all kidding aside, there are certain constitutions which seem to mate for life more readily than others. This does not mean that you should skip town on the first shuttle bus before sunrise, but it can be very informative to know what makes your mate tick.

His or her tendencies may drive you a little crazy and when you have a better understanding of what their typology tends towards, some empathy can prevail and a letting go can occur. When you realize that your *Calcarea carbonica* husband needs to sleep with a night-light on, you will know that it is because he suffers from significant fear of the dark. If you know your *Phosphorous* wife can be a little forgetful, you may understand if she has only picked up four of your five children after school ... or maybe not. When your *Sulphur* child refuses to wear shoes from May to October, you will know that they derive much of their energy from the earth and, like the roots of trees, they need to feel the soil between their toes.

IQ and EQ types can also make great bedfellows as their polarity can balance out the equation in a love relationship. An EQ type will provide growth, change and thrust to a relationship which can go on quite unbridled until her IQ soul mate shows up to gently impose his spherical, capping influence to help put form and structure to her ideas. It is a bit like the EQ Business Coach coming into an organization that has remained unchanged for years. She shakes the foundations; helping to effect change and then leaves it up to the IQ types to implement the structure.

On the same note, my two children, Jordan and Adie are a *Silicea* and *Phosphorous*, respectively. They recently set up mini-stores to sell their wares. Adie put up a sign to sell all her homemade beeswax candles for $30.00. Jordan suggested to her that she might do better to price them individually and that way she would make more money. At six, Adie had trouble seeing the merits of "making more money," but Jordan offered to sit and price them all for her and she went along with his suggestion in addition to better signage and positioning of her wares. Adie grew bored with the infinite level of detail and went to draw beautiful pictures of horses and then she subsequently sold them to Jordan for fair market value.

Siliceas tend to provide *Phosphorous* with the boundaries and structure that they grow to rely on to function well. *Phosphorous* provides *Silicea* with the spark needed for them to get out and experience things instead of staying home on the computer or with their nose in a book. *Pulsatillas* will love the *Lycopodium* who may be working hard all day climbing the corporate ladder and conversely *Lycopodium* will let their defences down at home and let the "little girl or boy" out to be effectively nurtured. Also, *Lycopodiums* will generally take good care of a *Pulsatilla*, who also needs to be charmed. In turn, they can feel quite fulfilled in their choice to remain at home to nurture the family

Calcarea carb provides their methodical approach to life which can help *Sulphur* to execute their inspirations. Admittedly, *Sulphur* can be one of the most challenging individuals to live with, so the easy-going affable characteristics of a *Calc* can withstand the daily, sometimes hourly, charge. And the *Calc* may feel less immovable as the Sulphur invokes excitement, change and thrust into the relationship.

The mating of spirit and earth pole constitutions probably have greater challenges, but I know of at least one awesome, refined *Silicea* woman who is madly in love with her exuberant *Sulphur* husband and they are very compatible. I was born a *Phosphorous*, but have found my soul mate to be a *Calcarea carbonica*, so while we benefit from the dichotomies of our relationship, we can also struggle like a tortoise and hare would if they shacked up together. He compares himself to a mild version of Woody Allen and I am more of a Kate Hepburn type.

My husband, Jeff, is very intellectual, grounded and loving. He is a doctor of homeopathic medicine and is writing a book on vaccinations and how effectively homeopathy can be used preventatively for families who choose not to use allopathic shots for immunity. The scope and nature of this kind of research and writing will probably take him some time, and he hopes to finish it within the next couple of years. Admittedly, I would have a tough time engaging in a project of this magnitude as I would get frustrated and want to move on.

When I first met Jeff, I was physically very cold from my waist down. If I put a hand on my abdomen, I literally felt frigid from having neglected my fertile, creative, sexual fire for over 15 years. Four years prior, I had taken a Hatha Yoga class and realized that I did not know how to breathe into that space down below the diaphragm. It was as if I had been panting for years, only filling my upper lungs superficially. When I first began to try to "belly breathe," I felt a profound fear as I tried to force air down into my neglected cavity. I became light-headed and dizzy as a result and wondered if a deeper natural rhythm would ever ensue.

It was interesting for me to meet someone that had the ability to make me laugh from the deepest place in my belly, naturally. As I felt myself trust and let go, I could feel my whole face and being opening up and emitting the juiciest laugh from the very basement of my soul. The laughter continued, and mysteriously, I felt embers of warmth sparking within my abdomen. These were coddled by a hermetic resonance which took off like a house on fire after we had formed our commitment. I had many dreams and images of many prior lifetimes together with Jeff. It felt as if I had come home.

At present, we are married, and we use our union to foster a strong relationship and commitment to our intimacy. This mutual celebration and honouring of our own divinity is really about tapping into a well-spring of energy that can be used to heal ourselves and nurture our own creativity. The approach we use is based very much on the research done by Mantak Chia who co-authored books such as, *The multi-Orgasmic Man*[17] and *Healing Love Through the Tao, Cultivating Female Sexual Energy.*[18]

As a result of living in resonance, I laugh often down to my loins, my belly is hot and I have no fear of deep sexual expression. It is interesting for me to note that as a result of these transformations, a couple of my colleagues have very recently typed me as a *"Sulph-a-podium"* which is a cross between *Sulphur and Lycopodium.* I am fascinated by this analogy as it means that I am effectively working on increasing my creative, generative capacity in a more conscious fashion. Crossing these imaginary "boundaries" from one pole to the other is a rarity, but it can be more easily done by working to achieve a state of health.

I find being aware of constitutions helps me to understand what makes others tick and understanding can help build tolerance. One day we were at a local restaurant and a very large woman was sitting alone at the next table and yelling loudly across the room to the staff in the kitchen telling them how much she enjoyed the soup. Her soupspoon was raised, as she was spouting its praises, and soup was dribbling over the side of the spoon onto her dress. Jordan was mortified for her and he elbowed me to say, "Mom, look at that woman, doesn't she know that she is embarrassing herself?" I replied, "No, I don't think so. She is a *Sulphur* and it is more important to her that she share how much she is enjoying her soup at this moment than how she might appear to others later on."

Jordan's refined nature and concern for how others perceive him made it difficult to empathize with the woman and I know he felt disgust for her. At 40, I thought she was awesome as her legs swung apart, back and forth on the barstool, and her wide smile and twinkling eyes exuded limitless mischievous energy. I am learning to let go of my inhibitions more and more, and I welcome these divine models!

CHAPTER 15

THE DEPTHS OF TREATMENT

I had spent most of my life looking outside myself for the source of my grief and anxiety. I spent a good deal of time blaming others for my own perceived misfortunes. I was so easily angered by anything that appeared to threaten my homemade suit of armour. I'd spent countless years and much energy arranging each shield of defence so that it would effectively protect my vital organs; my feelings. In fact, I wasn't sure what my true feelings were anymore as they were buried so far below the metal plates on the surface. Every reaction was filtered by the grief, anger, fear and guilt I harboured which skewed any of my real feelings when they would try to emerge. Sometimes I would listen to my reactions and wonder who the pathetic woman was that was speaking.

I honestly don't know what force urged me to continue with the remedies in those early days as I could feel every metal plate being unscrewed one agonizing turn at a time. This process was indeed destabilizing for me and the counter actions huge, and so from the onset when I began placing the single drop of the emotional remedies into two huge glasses of water I would try to suppress the fear as the black ogre in my imagination continued the intense ascent up over my head.

As mentioned, this lasted for almost three weeks when I noticed the muck and mire starting to subside. I felt a little bit better, a little more clear-headed and my energy level seemed somewhat increased from before. I embraced the opportunity to list all of my complaints for Patty who filled many sheets of blank paper over the months to follow. I remember reviewing all of my sufferings as if they happened yesterday, "…every winter I get three to four chronic sinus infections," I began, "wicked PMS lasting two weeks at a stretch, severe psoriasis on my scalp, monthly bladder and yeast infections, fogged-in every time there is a low pressure system, a constant hunger with bouts of over-eating and I'm dragged out exhausted all of the time."

When Patty recommended writing out a timeline before our next appointment, I went home to prepare this seemingly cerebral document for her reference. It hadn't occurred to me that I had never actually taken the events of my life and unravelled them one by one to present them like an entrée on paper before. I wrote about Jordan's traumatic delivery, my conversion to Judaism for marriage sake, my visits to the hospital emergency when I temporarily lost my vision due to stress, the mini-stroke suffered while taking the pill, the exploratory surgery when I suffered an inflamed bowel, the untimely death of my 43-year-old father by heart attack when I was 17, and my biological mother's suicide when I was eight.

After writing this all out, I remember shaking violently as if I was going into some sort of electrical shock, just from raising these long buried events to the surface like the bubbles in a glass of pop. Days afterwards, I was haunted by these memories and surprisingly, memories of many other minor shocks and traumas began to waken me at night or even while I was performing mundane tasks like cleaning a sink. These traumas attempted to consciously reveal their significance for this process. I recorded things like the years of being subjected to chlorine as a competitive swimmer, experimentation with recreational drugs in university, and my having lived with family and friends for weeks and sometimes months at a time during my biological mother's bouts of depression and schizophrenia.

I even had a couple of idiosyncrasies like washing my hands and brushing my teeth incessantly, even though my hands would bleed with the dryness during the winter months. In my youth, I wore exceedingly uncomfortable clothes; tight jeans with belts cinched to the tightest notch and hot athletic socks all summer long. I think now that this all must have been an effort to keep myself together in one emotional piece when inside I was really falling apart. The cleanliness, I'm sure, had much to do with the *"Syphilis"* running rampant through my genetic family tree.

Roger Morrison's *Desktop Guide to Keynotes and Confirmatory Symptoms*[19] is one of the best modern references to Homeopathic Materia Medica on the market and he does a great job of describing *Syphilis* in particular.

"In the *Syphilitic* miasm we see destructiveness on all levels but not a violent destruction – more like erosion. On the physical level, we see erosions of the bone; on the emotional level the patient may have a type of nihilism or a feeling to let everything crash down around him; and on the mental level we see a breakdown into insanity." Under the heading of "Mentals" he encapsulates some of the characteristics of this insidious disease, "Compulsive checking, compulsive hand washing, and fear of infection, disease, insanity and Alcoholism."[20]

I despise this disease more than any of the others. Imagine my eyes getting bigger and bigger as I poured over countless Materia Medicas finding significant symptomology in each to categorize the behaviour of many of my relatives. *Syphilis'* insidious, slow self-destructive nature can also be seen in many public figures in film and in politics. Marilyn Munroe and J.D. Salinger are both individuals who have displayed *Syphilitic* characteristics and I sympathize with friends and family who have had to witness their demise from creativity.

Fibromyalgia, the "condition" recently identified by traditional medicine, is really just an accumulation of symptoms which are mainly anchored to the miasm *Syphilis* and is easily annihilated through Heilkunst treatment. Dr. David Nye writes that, "The American College of Rheumatologists 1990 diagnostic criteria don't say that the aching has to be continuous, just chronic. You can hurt almost anywhere from FMS, not just in the 18 diagnostic tender points which were chosen because they are the most consistent from patient to patient."[21]

You can clearly see the thinking around how allopathic medicine renders diagnosis. First there has to be an authoritative body that legitimizes your symptoms and then they decide on the criteria which are most consistent from patient to patient. It appears we are literally sleepwalking if we allow this stumbling around in the dark as a rendering of diagnosis. Unfortunately, when these individuals find their way to the Heilkünstler's office, their condition has been exacerbated by iatrogenic (doctor induced) disease due to the barrage of drugs that only suppresses their pain, in addition to the 18 sore pressure points. Fibromyalgia is a relatively easy condition to cure. Their inner core can be surprisingly well, as measured by live blood cell analysis, as they're holding their emotional traumas in the fibrous tissue of the muscles. By using remedies to encourage the letting go of anger, grief, guilt and fear, their muscles relax and the chronic pain lifts.

Through the Hahnemann Center Clinic, I witnessed a patient whose spine was actually disintegrating; she eventually recovered sufficiently to leave her wheelchair. After three months, I met her at a health show and she was using a walker to get around. When I saw her six months later, she was walking with a cane. Her doctors had told her that she would never walk again.

If we keep using empirical thinking and simply naming or labelling diseases that arise in our midst, we threaten to compromise true diagnosis. We know that a disease will manifest in many different ways and will especially vary from person to person. The allopathic names just limit how the individual is perceived and thus treated. If one drug or a type of surgery worked for one person, then in all likelihood, it will do the same for another. This is a false premise guided solely by the intellect and we should look at fostering guiding principles that remain constant and allow a "unique" diagnosis to emerge from each individual. In 200 years, the principles of homeopathy have remained the same and no remedies have ever been recalled by their pharmaceutical companies compared with the Thalidomide catastrophe of the 1960s and the thousands of unrecorded deaths per year from correctly prescribed allopathic drugs. It is time to wake the sleepwalkers!

The next bout of remedies I received was for the delivery of each of my children. I remember having to call my mom to come over and look after the kids for a few hours as I was suffering abdominal cramping as part of the counter action to the remedy I told her that I was indeed passing blood far enough off the schedule of my normal menses that it was catching my attention. As this was still early in my treatment, my anger and frustration of having to endure this kind of discomfort was paramount. I also despaired about whether or not my health was truly getting better.

The next thing I was treated for was my conversion to Judaism. Up until recently I had always felt like some pawn in a rather sick game of chess. Even though I had some loose definition of my own spirituality, which did not resonate with any specific organized religion, and I considered myself a supporter of feminist principles, I still gave up the power of my convictions in order to acquiesce to what I thought was a stronger influence at the time. I chose authority over individuality.

Prior to the conversion, I didn't perceive that I had any strong sense of identity or community. So when I was asked about my unborn child's sense of community, I succumbed to the fear. The arguments in my mind continued, "Don't you want to become part of a rich heritage?" "What do you really have to offer in the way of an identity anyway?" The truth was I was in love, outnumbered and their arguments were more convincing than mine... I just didn't realize what I might be losing in the process. When I first saw Patty, I was still in the throes of a significant identity crisis. I had chosen to please my in-laws to the point of loss of self and I needed to address the residual anger and grief.

Back in the 1980s during university, flitting from jobs in bars, modeling and finally settling into a clerical job with the federal government, I experienced a rash of minor illnesses that often saw me at the emergency room of the local hospital. I had an inflamed bowel that was detected during a laparoscopy, lost my sight to the point of tunnel vision during a stress attack, and once had a minor stroke due to taking the birth control pill. I lived with my aunt and uncle in Toronto. They were both alcoholics, with enough of their own hot baggage to keep a mental ward hopping.

I ducked empty drink glasses thrown at my aunt by my uncle. I avoided my uncle's attempts to sexually accost me on countless occasions. And my aunt would arrange for me to attend plays and operas while she spent the evening in a hotel room with her lover. I willingly debriefed her on the content of the performances in order to protect her from being found out. Ironically, I attribute much of my exposure to culture from these years.

My aunt was my biological mother's sister who also shared my unique gene pool. She died of a mysterious cancer the week Jordan was born. Her neck blew up with a grapefruit-like tumour and she was gone within about five months. It was sad when she lost her voice as she loved to talk and she spent hours just lunching with friends. I sent her favourite, yellow roses, just before she died. I still missed the fun she and I would have traveling, eating out at swanky restaurants and late night chats on the yacht we lived on in the summer months.

I know that I was beginning to sustain some of the impact from the issues that plagued my family and like any other red blooded North American I went looking for relief from doctors. They analyzed me and parceled me off in parts to psychologists, specialists and internists. Most of the psychologists were sicker than I. One psychiatrist I saw at the University of Toronto, while I was a student there, had an abnormal way of leering, and when he rubbed his hands continuously at the second appointment, I bolted from the chair and out of his office never to return.

As mentioned earlier, in 1981 my father, the youngest of six surviving children with no apparent history of heart disease, died at the age of 43 of a heart attack. To me, it was apparent that he needed to be with my mother who was the love of his life. I think it is interesting to note that after receiving *Natrum Muriaticum* (the remedy used to treat grief) during this point in my time line, I developed canker sores all over my bottom lip in my mouth, the severest case of psoriasis around the perimeter of my scalp, and intense stitches of pain in my chest. These were all key symptoms of this remedy profiled in the homeopathic books I was researching on my own. Even my emotional issues were effectively following the direction of cure, from the inside out to the surface!

I once asked Patty, "How does a real bona fide healthy person react when they are ill?" She immediately responded, "Why they look within to heal themselves, of course, detecting the imbalances before they become disease. Illness is a product of our evolution and we need to identify why we have energetically resonated with the disease in the first place. A classroom full of kids may be exposed to the mumps, but only a few will get it. Why is that? Identifying the true reason for the disease at the root level of initial resonance is as important as taking the correct remedy through proper diagnosis."

What a concept! Yet I was only getting brief glimmers of how I might one day be capable of doing this for myself. For now, I relied very heavily on those who effectively supported me and I read every recommended resource on Homeopathy like a fiend. As I got closer to those really "big" events on my timeline, Patty gave me the number of her private line next to her bed. I only used this number once as I continued to shed another piece of the armour.

At this point in my timeline, things began to flip for me emotionally. I began to take more ownership for my issues and I began to reap some of the benefits emerging out of my arduous journey. I used other sources of support during my treatment like chiropractic care and also hands-on cranial sacral therapy. I had a very positive experience with a "hands-on healer" during a cranial sacral session and without going into too much detail, I'll just quote a couple of paragraphs from the account I wrote some time later:

All of a sudden I sensed energy rushing forcefully into my body. It was the purest essence of love and joy I had ever felt. This was the most indescribable sensation I'd ever had. It felt as if the vessel, that was my body, could not contain all of the energy pouring into me and I felt myself arch my back slightly off the table in an attempt to provide a conduit for it to flow. The purpose of the energy was to express love, without any of the usual earthly binds, and connect me with a universal knowingness. The tears poured soundlessly and effortlessly down the sides of my cheeks as a means to address the overflowing sensations.

On some level I felt myself look to see the source of this energy. I use the word look, but I'm not sure I ever opened my eyes. I did, however, see the most incredible white light coming through the ceiling and into the core of my stomach. The make-up of this light was extraordinary. It was a wide column almost a foot and a half in diameter composed of particles of dancing, shimmering, white and silver all headed towards the centre of my body.

After the light receded somewhat, and the sensations were reduced to a more normal level, I returned to focus on my breathing and my more 'earthly state of being.' The healer turned the dimmer switch up enough so that I could see her standing beside me. She looked over at me and asked if I was all right. Not knowing what she may have perceived during my experience with the light, I shakily answered that I was fine. I have not forgotten, or will ever forget, the exact words she said next, "Allyson, I have a message for you from the Universe. Your mother loves you very much and wants you to know that you are very much connected to something greater than the realm of your day-to-day living. Furthermore she wants to remind you that, your children will always have this knowingness because you are their mother and you are her daughter."

The healer did not know that my mother had died as this was my first session with her and there was no reason to have told her beforehand. As stated earlier, my mother died in 1971, by her own hand, when I was eight years old. Her father was committed for the rest of his life to a mental institution before my mother's eighth birthday. I know I don't need to illustrate any further the source of my genetic issues or my fear around contracting elements of this disease. I know that one of my main missions during this lifetime was to cure this miasmic influence for myself and for my children. The buck would stop here and my inherited landmines were to be defused!

Through treatment, it was becoming clearer to me that I was unequivocally on the path to cure. As difficult and daunting as this journey was proving to be, given my profound healing reactions that sometimes lasted weeks, with resounding messages from truer a source than I had ever perceived, I forged on. I was continually amazed at how imperative it was for my psyche to catch up in awareness to what was occurring in my physical body. My body only seemed to physically heal once I effectively figured out what the intended piece of "knowing" was. This was curing from the inside out and there was no going back.

Once the issue was unlocked, I walked through a door and out the other side. Symptoms were truly being annihilated permanently.

I sometimes looked jealously to my family and friends who were also going through treatment and only seemed to experience a headache for a day or two before seemingly moving past their related issues with each remedy. It seemed I had been avoiding many hard-core issues and I was speeding up my personal evolution a hundred-fold. I had a ton of work to do.

I have a theory that each person's healing reaction is based on how close or how far they have ventured off their intended karmic path. Each one of us has intentions that we are mandated to fulfill before incarnating into a lifetime. Surprisingly, our lives aren't just a random act of meaningless transgressions. Each of us has a contract to fulfill and disease was born as a function of reminding us of that purpose.

At birth, our memory of this contract with the divine is erased, similar to when God kicked us out of the Garden of Eden. However, if we work hard at becoming truly conscious solely for ourselves, we can get back to this tree of knowledge through health and well-being in a true sense. The tree of knowledge is really a big cosmic library entitled the "Akashic Records" by some mystics. I knew I was beginning to tap into a source of knowledge greater than what my limited diseased psyche could have developed over my misguided lifetime.

Thorwald Dethlefsen, who wrote *The Healing Power of Illness*[22] states that our sole mission during each of our lives is to become conscious. Illness just provides us with an opportunity to accomplish this effectively by focusing our attention on the affection. And if we're not paying attention, the symptoms just get stronger and more obvious until we do. We've all heard of people who have changed their lifestyle and thought processes and as a result have gone into "spontaneous remission."

Our life paths can be represented by an elastic band that sometimes becomes stretched on a path of unconscious ill intent. If we sway too far from our inner truth, the counter action brought on by taking the remedy will drive us back closer to where we are destined to be, fulfilling our contract with the divine.

We just have to know how to pay attention and interpret the road signs. If we don't watch carefully, the answers will appear in our symptoms.

By using the system of Heilkunst, we short circuit the potentiality for disease and become more conscious. The system of Heilkunst will open the doors, but it is entirely our choice whether we walk through them.

Narayan-Singh wrote *Messages From The Body*,[23] which is a reference book I used often during my own treatment. He effectively matches body symptoms with the soul-spiritual meaning. He wrote, "Everything begins and ends in consciousness, and the body is a kind of 'last ditch defence' arena regarding the consciousness problem that is precipitating the disturbance. Something is awry in our consciousness, and our body has 'taken the rap' for us to let us know that this 'delusional-illusional' process cannot continue any more."

I loved how my children would call the remedies, "memories" as this is actually a more accurate rendering in my mind. Each remedy is an energetic memory of its animal, plant or mineral source. Jordan quickly began to catch on to what was contained in each of the little dropper bottles prescribed for him and he would say, "Today I'm feeling angry, Mommy, I need the anger memory!" And like a little bird he would open his mouth and wait for me to dispense the drop onto his tongue.

When Jordan was five years old, he came home with a picture of a policeman. He had blackened the face violently with red and black crayon. I jokingly thought I had a potential mini-anarchist on my hands and I gently questioned his intent behind the drawing. When I asked Jordan what was in his mind when he was colouring the picture, he answered, "I just wanted to try on Sam's anger memory to see how it feels." Sam was a classmate of his who was typed with ADHD.

The meaningful "occurrences" in my life began to multiply. One time, at a cottage, while telling a friend about my natural mom and describing all the things she loved, I was in the midst of telling her that my mom's favourite colour was red/orange. I was saying to my friend that, "Crayola crayons had a red/orange crayon and I don't even know if Crayola has actually labelled this crayon any differently to this day. I used to colour pictures for her predominantly using this colour. I'll never forget how she used to buy roses, or a scarf or lipstick of this particular hue." Just at that precise moment, a Monarch Butterfly landed on the mesh screen of the window where we were sitting. It was 10:30 at night and it occurred to me that I had never before seen a butterfly in flight so late in the evening. This butterfly remained on the screen for my viewing pleasure for two whole days!

I even asked my husband if he could go out and check to see if she was alive and not somehow caught in the mesh of the screen. At six feet two inches, he was barely able to reach her delicate body with a fishing rod, but he gently pried her off the screen. She hung, suspended momentarily in mid air before she fluttered back to the same spot to remain another whole day. The red/orange of the Monarch was the exact colour I was trying to describe to my friend.

The kids love when I tell this story to them and it has been rather embarrassing at times. Once we went to see a butterfly exhibit at a local greenhouse and when a Monarch fluttered above the greenery over head, both kids screamed excitedly, "Mom, it's your mom! Look she has come here to visit you!" Well, I can tell you the looks from passers-by were pretty interesting and I smiled weakly at Jordan and Adie in agreement. For the next hour or so, in that greenhouse, a great many butterflies landed on both the kids. People were amazed at their obvious attraction as none of these winged nymphs ever landed on anyone else while we were there.

Another time, the kids and I were stuck in traffic on the freeway, talking about my mom. Jordan wanted to know if there was a possibility that Adie was my mom reincarnated. I answered that I didn't know, and he was pressing me about what date my mom died and how long it normally takes spirits to find a new body to jump into and just as Adie proudly announced that her middle name is Valerie, after her grandmother, a Monarch sailed by the windshield of the car. The conversation stopped dead, like the traffic, as we watched this majestic being flutter by unhurried and unbridled. Both kids yelled, "See we told you mom, Adie is your Mom!" What could I say to that?

During this journey into Heilkunst, I logged many of these "cosmic coincidences" and I celebrate every time I am attuned and healthy enough to recognize them as the gifts that they are. They may have always occurred in my life; however, I did not possess the organs to effectively see them in my former numb state of being.

As a result of taking my vaccination remedies I experienced the following healing crises which lasted for six months and which I'll illustrate through an e-mail I wrote to Patty at the time:

I'm experiencing some very significant pain in my upper back and neck. I have a pinched nerve in my neck, knots of muscle spasms on both sides of my spine (worse on the right), a rib keeps popping out which provides exquisite pain, and it feels as if I'm unable to support my weight and my vertebrae are being crushed together. I feel as if my chest is caving in and I'm unable to take a full breath without pain...and this shallow apnea is frustrating as it leaves me feeling very unfulfilled. An oncoming sneeze is terrifying!

I'm trying to get to the gym 2-3 times a week to gently increase the strength in my muscles in that region. Arnica, Ruta, and Rhus Tox, haven't touched it, and my chiropractor says I'm a complete mess. I'm so knotted up that 10 minutes worth of adjustments on just the one area only holds for up to an hour or so afterwards. I'm using a hot water bottle, a hand held massager, Tylenol and even resorted to an allopathic muscle relaxant for the first time tonight.

It is interesting to me that it was at this point that I gave up my lucrative consulting job with the federal government to write poetry, articles for holistic publications, and short works of fiction. Entire pieces of prose were coming to me in dreams and visions again, just like when I was a child. I would be folding laundry or vacuuming and a piece would start writing itself in my head. I would stop everything I was doing just to jot it down. And once I made the decision to serve this fiery muse from within, the pain in my neck and back disappeared almost instantaneously. The ability to hear my inner voice had been reawakened through my treatment. After the experience with the silver and white light creativity began to seep slowly back into my life and I allowed it. As I began to let go a tiny bit more, I asked, "Where was I headed now?"

CHAPTER 16

MY BIRTH

Taking the remedies for the trauma sustained from my own birth brought some very interesting sensations as described in an article I was asked to write for the Hahnemann College periodical, *The Heilkunst Journal:*[24]

This week, I've just gone through my birth. My lungs have mysteriously filled with water, I passed black muconium-like stool for two days, and I developed a very pronounced red mark shaped like Australia on my forehead. The cool part was that I felt as if I'd been pushed through the neck of a pop bottle. The only way I can describe the sensation on the other side is like when the Starship Enterprise has just 'warped' from one galaxy to arrive in another. The engines are in neutral as I take in the star-filled cosmos, coasting on a sea of tranquility. I feel as if I'm vibrating at a different frequency – actually two frequencies. One part of me is so solidly connected to the earth where I'm now resonating with a sense of peace and inner watchfulness that I have never felt before.

This had been such a surprising and incredible journey thus far. I'd gone through traumatic and daunting healing crises where I felt I had actually spent a day "in labour" during the homeopathic cleansing for the trauma of my daughter's birth. I'd had my scalp break out with psoriasis, cold sores in my mouth and pains in my chest while revisiting my father's death. And that was just the physical stuff! The anger I experienced would have enabled me to rip the door off a saloon in a Spaghetti Western and start a mean bar room brawl. During my vaccinations, I was paralyzed with pain from my chest up to the base of my skull.

It is also interesting to note that I had shifted constitutions. I was responding much more as a *Phosphorous* now, whereas, as a *Pulsatilla* I was always in a state of emotional angst, requiring a constant flow of love and adoration from outside that was not always forthcoming. This tendency proved to be self-nihilistic during my teens and early 20s as I was not always capable of discerning the integrity of the source. As a *Phosphorous*, I felt more lightness of being and have since returned to the characteristic playfulness reminiscent of my early childhood before my mother died.

One part of me felt a truer, more profound connection to the earth and cosmos and a psychic energy that feeds my being with pure love, a sense of wonderment and context. I was not going to be running off to the local yogic ashram with some new mystical sense of self but I felt a more grounded wonder and principled knowing. I have seemingly fallen from grace many times in my life, including entertaining desires to end it all. Looking back, I was always caught before the final moment by a sense of inner purpose that sparked an ember that I was able to derive the tiniest flame from.

More importantly, my connection to the earth, where all the black ooze, grief and fear used to reside is now the primary source for my own love and creativity. My cranial sacral therapist at the time suggested I "hug more trees" to remain more grounded to the earth during my more mystical phases. Earlier, I had desired to remain closer to the cosmic pole in order to avoid descending into the black pit of the earth pole. Now the earth turned out to be the source of my real power and strength. Through this process, I was experiencing a kind of re-birth and this newly found energy was big and awe inspiring. But I was not healthy enough yet to know how to effectively play with my new psychic toys. It was sort of like receiving a radio station from Russia without an interpreter. My life became a gift of flight and I marvelled at my un-harnessed desire for exploration. The armour was now flying off at an alarming rate and the plates could be heard crashing to the ground one after another.

As I looked toward my remaining journey into the genetic miasms, I imagined five office towers looming before me. If it was going to be similar to the way I'd experienced sequential treatment so far, I was sure to shed a layer of skin like a snake during the dance with all psoric skin disease, I may even cough up a lung during the tubercular phase and by the time I hit *Syphilis*, I should be enjoying my stay at "Shady Acres" convalescing and hugging a variety of trees with great abandon. I expected the most profound reaction to this last remedy given the self-destructive patterning that runs rampant through my mother's family.

I playfully imagined that if I were to explain my tumultuous journey thus far through physical and emotional traumas towards insight and health to someone like Jean Luc Picard of the Star Ship Enterprise (his character might even be one of the few people who would not think I was crazy), and tell him of the daunting miasmic feats ahead of me; I'm sure he would say the same thing he always does to his partner in cosmic adventuring, "Make it so, Number 1, make it so!"

CHAPTER 17

THE MIASMS

D r. Samuel Hahnemann noted that while many of his patients were experiencing a cure, there were others who had a return of their old symptoms. Based on his research and meticulous clinical trials, he knew that the system of medicine, law of similars, was sound. He also knew there was something that he had overlooked.

Rudolf Verspoor wrote in *The Dynamic Legacy: From Homeopathy to Heilkunst* about Hahnemann's discovery: "He realized that the treatment to date based on the prevailing symptoms, did not constitute a full cure; there remained hidden diseases not visible in any symptoms. He knew that the problem lay not in the lack of known medicines but in his lack of knowledge of disease."[25]

In essence, what Hahnemann figured out was that there were constant diseases lying quietly dormant at the core of every individual. If a person sustained enough strains, stresses and traumas over the course of their lifetime, then the sleeping miasms would awaken to rear their ugly heads.

The miasms have become a fundamental aspect of Heilkunst. These are primary, constant diseases that have remained with us over thousands of years.

While chronic and infectious in nature, they can also be passed down from one generation to another. By the early 1800s, Hahnemann had discovered three chronic miasms: *Psora, Sycosis* and *Syphilis.*

Simply put, *Psora* has been described as the "itch disease" and affects our largest surface organs of all, the skin and lungs, stemming from biblical times. Psora, from the Hebrew word "tsorat," was often used to denote leprous conditions. Eczema, psoriasis and scabies stem from this constant unwavering disease.

Hahnemann identified *Sycosis* by the small common genital warts which reminded him of figs in their shape and texture. The Greek word for fig is sycosis. It originally comes from a gonorrheal infection and leads to anxiety, aggressiveness and excesses of behaviour.

Roger Morrison types these individuals as, "excessively passionate people who are led to problems from strong needs for expression of the passion." They are extremists drawn to excesses in their relationships, their vices and their sexuality.

Syphilis is represented by the characteristic genital ulcer. On the surface, there can be marked tissue destruction and degeneration, but in essence the more corrosive effects are found in the mind. Suicide, ritualistic behaviours, serious mental disorders and addictions can stem from the core of this chronic miasm.

As we have evolved beyond Hahnemann's time, we have identified two more of these constant diseases to be tuberculosis and cancer. Tuberculosis was realized by Hahnemann's followers and identified as "pseudo-*Psora*" until later in the 19th century when tuberculosis emerged as a full-fledged illness in Europe. A homeopath by the name of Compton Burnett in England made a "nosode" of the disease by extracting the sputum of an infectious tubercular patient. Like cures exactly like!

Based on natural law, "nosodes" are made into homeopathic remedies through dilution and succession (smack a small bottle of water against the palm of your hand and watch for the vortex, a mini-tornado of energy!) and fed back to a patient with the same disease. Voilà, a cure!

Tuberculosis patients are restless, unfulfilled, romantic types who desire change and travel. They can also be caustic in nature and suffer allergies and dislikes to furred animals. Like *Syphilis*, they can also suffer from compulsive, ritualistic behaviours.

The essence of cancer is sensitivity. These patients live "outside" themselves, attempting to avoid "the eye of the storm" so to speak. If you ask them how they are, they will often tell you about their husband or children. They are sensitive to the plights of the world and suffer criticism badly. Their anxiety is for others and events generally. These patients are obsessed with news and world effects and do not wholly embrace their own lives.

Carcinosin is fastidious and worse from consolation. They desire chocolate, have a love of dancing and they are exhilarated by thunderstorms. It is also a great remedy for opposites; there can be great love or desire, then intense hate or aversion. Other homeopaths have cited that cancer is the ultimate penalty for the unlived life, and Wilhelm Reich, who spent his life dedicated to researching the treatment of cancer using Orgone energy, saw it as a process of contraction of the life energy. It is no wonder that a cancer patient's cells transform from largely a potassium base to a saline base and their PH levels drop from alkaline to acid. This is representative of the overall sclerotic effect of disease. Hahnemann called cancer the "wasting disease" as patients lose a great deal of weight and waste away slowly over time.

Every one of us carries latent chronic miasms. Whether we manifest symptoms of the disease or not during the course of a lifetime, we carry them unknowingly in our genetic code as gifts for our children who may succumb to the disease. Manifestation of symptoms based on these dormant roots is determined by the load we are carrying and the amount of stress and strain we invoke in our lives. The disease will invoke a "state of mind" long before the symptoms manifest. Someone with a *Tuberculinum* miasm will have a stronger predisposition for lung infections such as bronchitis, whooping cough and pneumonia. The *Tuberculinum* state of mind is characterized by restlessness, romantism and yearning individuals characterized well in the French movie

Amelie. As mentioned earlier, the only possibility of curing chronic miasms is by applying natural law, the law of similars.

More recently, research at The Hahnemann Center Clinic in Ottawa, Canada, is unearthing two more miasms, *Malaria* and *Ringworm*. During my fifth round of miasms, I was one of the fortunate patients to exhibit symptoms for both these latent diseases. Based on where I am in my miasmic journey; about five or six generations back into my ancestry, there must have been relatives who were bitten by an infected mosquito or contracted ringworm and I was lucky enough to have manifested their symptoms for treatment. The loop is now closed. Finally!

CHAPTER 18

MY MIASMIC BAGGAGE

This was the part of the voyage that I feared the most. If the bulk of what I had sustained over my lifetime was rooted here, then I was in for healing reactions of tsunami proportions. This was where the ancestral baggage was going to be unleashed into the fray of my being. How would all that mental illness filter out of me without claiming my psyche en route?

During my lifetime, I had a certain degree of understanding and empathy for the choices I had made in relation to the traumas I had sustained. In many cases, I was aware of the conscious choices I had made. I knew that I ended up at the hospital emergency room for loss of vision because I could no longer bear "seeing"my present reality. I knew I had great difficulty with my periods because I held so much grief and I could not effectively surrender to my own femininity. I knew that I had not effectively separated from my mother after she died. Grief and anger manifested in the chronic sinus, bladder and bronchial infections I had treated with countless prescriptions of antibiotics.

However, the miasms were completely uncharted territory and I was going to have to surrender to a process I did not yet comprehend. My fiery will helped me to overcome the fear I did not allow to surface which left my ability to trust and surrender lopsided and clueless. I had no idea how to let go as trauma had only taught me how to effectively hang on and will my way through everything like a bull at an English high tea party!

The thing I had not lent enough credence to yet was that I was a whole lot healthier than at the onset of treatment. Almost all of my physical symptoms and ailments were gone and I did feel more grounded, aware and stronger on all levels. I wondered if my level of consciousness had grown enough to accept the responsibility of the inner work I still needed to do. In essence, I had no choice if I wanted to potentially clean the slate of ancestral debris for my self and my children.

Secretly, I began to pretend I was dancing with my arch nemesis, disease, as I demanded that she, "Bring it on, I dare ya!" What else was I to do, but position myself for a full frontal attack? At least assuming this stance made me feel like I was invoking my will! Like in the movie *The Matrix*, I had already swallowed the red pill and there was no turning back. I could only hope that when I reached Zion, something would be left after the imminent destruction.

At this stage, I also began to suspect that the remedies had a dual purpose. One stream involved the physical and emotional ramifications of the remedy I had taken. The other showed what I needed to accomplish to fulfill obligations over this and other lifetimes. I felt as if I was speeding up my karma and paying down debts faster than before.

In essence, I began to realize that my outer world was nothing more than an increasingly clearer reflection of my inner world. I had one responsibility and that was to my own inner world. This took my area of influence and responsibility down to a very manageable level. The healthier I became, the more I focused in on me. Like a drop in a pool of water, ripples of negativity with family or friends seemed to shift based on the changes I was making to this newfound thing I was getting to know as "self." Many of my relationships had been constructed out of my need to rescue others, and as I found less reason to provide this martyrdom service to others, these one-sided relationships dropped off. Miraculously, these people seemed to land more squarely on their own two feet and were finally able to find their own way. My support to them was such a dis-service as it short-circuited their ability to find their own true potential. I was allopathically impinging on their personal direction of cure. This also made room for more resonant authentic truth-seekers in my own life.

I also had to come to the realization that I deserved health. What a concept! Formerly, I didn't know what I didn't know and now I was beginning to live full time apart from *The Matrix*. I was using my "visitor's pass" to the "outside" less and learning more about my own inner Zion. Looking back I could see my one-way collision course toward self-annihilation. The efforts had been huge and my payoff minimal. I manipulated and muscled every domain I entered in my efforts to control what was never mine to control. Suppressing the shadow was definitely a full-time job. If I could see this for myself, what did this mean for the rest of humanity? I had to suppress the old desire to tell everyone I knew about what I was learning. Once, when I did try to explain what I was living to a close family member, she suggested that she would rather die than sustain the healing reactions that I had had.

What she didn't realize was that she is living in the realm of sacrifice. The drugs, the numbness and the fear are not freedom in any form. Even gangrene settles in the extremities in order to save your vital core. I had lost nothing in my healing reactions but my diseases, and gained the responsibility of consciousness. And many of the people I love were having none of it! I took the remedy for grief and worked harder at letting my need for their health go and continued on my one sole responsibility toward cure.

Shortly after taking *Psorinum*, I adopted pneumonia-like symptoms. As my lungs filled up with water I took a moment to write an e-mail to Patty:

> *I'm feeling my mother's pain as she made the choice to go into the enclosed garage and turn on the car to take her final breaths before her death. Patty, I actually feel like I'm dying in my own skin and that this loss is too hard to bear any longer. I also feel the abandonment of not only her death, but of every single individual I've ever felt love and support from who I have left.*

I told my husband about an image I kept getting of a body of water that lies at the very core of my being and how the water was churning, kicking up tidal waves, trying to drown me from the inside out. Any conduit to the surface would do. Tear ducts, nostrils, breath, even my sweat and urine felt rancid and thick with the pain.

I was sipping at my water, which contained the remedies for grief, anxiety, fear, anger and congestion. I truly feared that this time I might die from this. My breathing became very shallow as my lung capacity diminished. I felt as if I was drowning from the inside out! In essence, a part of me was indeed dying so that a rebirth of sorts could take place.

After reading my e-mail Patty and Rudi called me that same night. I realized that I must have caught their attention when I heard them both on the line, conference style. I tried to express further, in shallow breaths, exactly what I was feeling. During consultations, Patty always managed to hear something indicative in my plights, some fundamental message relayed from a source I was not always aware of. This intuitive aspect of Heilkunst is key to rendering a true diagnosis which is effectively taught and integrated in this art of medical science. However, I'll never forget how angry I was at Rudi, at the time, for suggesting that I had to let go of my mother in order to move through this healing reaction. Why didn't he just ask me to push Mount Everest to the left an inch or two? That would have been much easier.

Two nights later I woke to a vision of lying on the front seat of the car with my mother that fateful day in the garage, the engine was running and she was telling me it was time for us to go. She began her ascent, rising above me, beckoning for me to follow her. Seconds seemed to tick by. Then the next thing I heard was a scream, "NNNOOOOOOOOOOOOOOO." It was my own voice and I was running to the outside of the garage to suck pure oxygen into very congested lungs. I woke up with a jolt, attempting to breathe, wheezing and coughing.

I knew in that moment that my mother had taken part of me with her on that day in September. In 29 years I had never separated that part of myself from her destiny. I had so loved my mother and she was the person I had always keenly identified with. In fact, she was still defining me for almost 30 years. I can now understand the choice I made at the time to send part of my psyche with her out of love, desperation and grief. I had never adopted my own true ego as the grief kept me wrapped up so intrinsically with her, locked in the past. By sucking in the pure air for myself, and making this new choice to live for the first time in my life, I effectively separated my karmic journey from hers. It was up to her to take possession for her own choice as it was not mine any more. Upon coming to this realization, a drain seemed to open, and my lungs cleared completely within 12 hours.

I felt as if a whole new sense of health was now awakening within me; a monumental birth of self in a real way, with a truer integrity. I felt I claimed my existence for the first time and I felt a profound inner celebration. I had no idea I had sold part of myself off to death to be with her. Before now, I was never really a fully operational model with a whole ego of my own.

I was amazed at how this vortex towards health kept spiraling up from the muck and mire of disease. It had defined so many aspects of my existence. I had gone along trying to address one symptom at a time thinking that they are independent agents without any roots. I have never suffered a sinus or lung infection from that day to this.

Narayan Singh offers that lung problems are due to "suffering from depression and chronic grief because they are deeply afraid of taking in life energy. They feel unworthy of living fully, and they are alone, sad and non-belonging, with no sense of acceptance."[26] I know that these clinical observations were true for me.

At each juncture on my Heilkunst map, I wrestled with the demons that were becoming increasingly clearer offshoots of the roots entangled below the surface. More and more, I stopped letting them define me and more armour dropped to the side. I needed less protection from the outside world. I could trust myself more to honour my inner needs as opposed to being defined by others' expectations. I was living more in the moment and less in the past. I started to feel empowered to actively employ my own sword of truth to hack away at each tendril. I could see them reaching for me in old patterns and I was starting to see clearly who their parents were!

As a child, every year when served my birthday cake, I'd make one simple wish,

"Please God, just let me realize some measure of peace in this lifetime." I could now say that I felt true peace for the first time in my life. I silently gave thanks to those I felt I owed karmic credit to: my awesome son Jordan who led me to the medicine, Patty Smith for her warmth and understanding of the system of medicine, Rudi and Steven, a couple of amazing researchers who boldly went where no man or woman had gone before, and Dr. Samuel Hahnemann's impeccable genius. With what I had gleaned thus far, I was gaining the courage "To Be" and I embarked on a higher potency of the miasms starting with *Psora* and ending at *Syphilinum*!

CHAPTER 19

ROUND NUMBER TWO

B y the second year of treatment, I was working for the Hahnemann College for Heilkunst, HCH, as their registrar. I also began to embark on my own studies to become a physician. I remember it was the Monday after the 2001 Canadian Conference of National United Professional Association of Trained Homeopaths (NUPATH) in Toronto. I was completely exhausted. Over the last 15 days, I'd either worked or been in-class. As I backed the van up across the lawn to the front door of the Hahnemann College, I thought about how I was just going to do what I could today to get the conference materials put away and some of the financial fall out from the conference taken care of. I was dressed in jeans and a sweatshirt and my hair was still damp from the shower. This was going to be my day just to putter with the necessities.

Jordan was in the back of the van and I asked him to help me with some of the smaller boxes before I dropped him off at school. He said, "No thanks" and continued to play with his computer game. I felt raw and numb as I dragged the boxes out of the back and lugged them over the threshold into the main classroom to the cupboards beyond. I had also fasted since midnight as I was scheduled for my live blood analysis follow-up in half an hour, the emptiness in my belly chiding me to fill it with rest and food which is not what I had planned for the day.

With Jordan delivered to school, I headed back to work and the HCH Clinic for my appointment. I kept reminding myself that I had arranged to take this coming Friday off. It would be the first day entirely devoted to me in almost three months. I had visions of a hot bath and a delicious book other than *The Dynamic Legacy: From Homeopathy to Heilkunst.*

I parked the car and made my way up the front steps. The Live Blood Analysis was performed in the same building I worked in along with five other Heilkunstler physicians. I looked forward to seeing what had transpired since I'd made some regimenal changes over the last six weeks. I was also aware that I should relish the half hour I'd carved out for myself to explore this facet of myself.

As I stepped into the front foyer, a prospective student who I'd spent some time talking to at the NUPATH conference greeted me. She and her mother, who were visiting from Europe, were in town for the conference and unbeknownst to me, they were waiting to meet with me in addition to having a tour of the Clinic. Because the student was from out of town, I couldn't very well ask her to come back at a more convenient time. I let them know that I would be happy to meet with her after I had my appointment and they should make themselves comfortable until then.

I was finally settled into my practitioner's office and we were just going over my blood cell improvements when a knock came at the door. One of the physicians had fielded a call from my sister-in-law, in Toronto, who wanted to speak with me. The physician was not aware that I was in a formal consultation, and quickly realized that she should just take a message on my behalf.

Despite my level of exhaustion, I saw significant improvements in my blood analysis and I left her office to meet with the student as my stomach reminded me of its own plight. The student and I discussed the program and she proceeded to translate, almost verbatim, everything to her mother in her mother tongue. I was wondering what the purpose of this was as I know the mother was not interested in pursuing studies with us. So I sat patiently during the intervals it took for her to illustrate the details of the program in German.

The meeting finally concluded, and I went to my office to pick up the morning phone calls and to return the call to my sister-in-law. When I reached her, she very excitedly reported that she was coming to visit us for four days on this Thursday. Despite the fact that I stated that this wasn't a particularly good time for me, and in fact during the conversation, I even ventured to say the word, "no," she was coming anyway. She reminded me that I had encouraged her into Heilkunst treatment and she had gone ahead and booked the time off work. She was coming and that was that. I could see my hot bubble bath turning to molten lava as my blood began to boil.

When I tried to make her aware of my plans, she said that she had no intention of interfering with my time to myself and that we could just spend the day chatting and reading in the same house. Over the past year or so, she had spent hour after hour picking my weary brain on the subject of Heilkunst to try and allay her own fears in an effort to embark on her own journey. I had a pretty good idea how Friday would shape up for her and it wasn't remotely close to how I wanted to spend the day.

Another knock came at my door and the prospective student asked if she could ask me a few more questions. Once again I fielded them the best I could and the translation continued. By this time, I was feeling weak and sick to my stomach. I finally excused myself, explaining the situation, and I literally fled the building close to tears. I drove to a local deli for a bagel and a rare coffee. To heck with the regimen, I thought!

As I sat in the restaurant, I tried to take stock of my present circumstances. I was wondering why I wasn't able to just focus on what I needed to do for myself. This was such an old pattern of how easily I always get diverted from my own path into the realm of what everyone else wanted. Like the *Pulsatilla* flower I was, at this time, I seemed to waft in the winds of everyone else's desires. God, how I hated my life in that defining moment! I wondered what would happen if I just turned the car south towards New Mexico and just kept driving.

As I left the deli, I remembered that I had a package waiting for me to pick up at the post office for the HCH. As I turned into the parking lot of the post office, I almost ran over a woman on the sidewalk. She looked up startled like a deer in the headlights. I swerved to avoid hitting her, just as I recognized her face. She was a woman I used to carpool with when I worked in a government office over a year ago. She had spent hours as we drove mornings and evenings, droning on about her two teenage daughters and I stupidly spent the same hours trying to give useless advice by empathetically illustrating what I thought was her children's plight. By some mercy, she did not recognize me and I continued into the post office avoiding what would have been yet another drain on my depleted energy level. The day's occurrences were beginning to form a theme.

As I returned to my car, I tried to think of some little thing I could do to feed my soul on the way back to the office. My favourite consignment shop was en route and a new shirt might help lift my spirits. I was browsing the racks and located something in basic black. "Like cures like," right?!!! As I went to pay for the item at the cash I looked up into the face of a woman I had gone to high school with. In fact she had been a friend until she had been intimate with my boyfriend in my parents' bed while we were away in Florida for vacation. My advice still remains, "Don't ask untrustworthy *Sulphur* boyfriends of three years to feed your cats while you're away on the gulf coast!" Please don't ask me how we knew, except that my parents could not use those sheets again.

I could see that she recognized me and that she was searching the recesses of her brain for the link. As it registered, the embarrassment also coloured her face a luscious rose. I said hello as evenly as I could for a woman unravelling before her eyes. She attempted to erase the memory from her face and smiled back at me. We talked for a moment about what became of friends we once had in common. Purposefully, the *Sulphur* beau never came up in the conversation.

As I got back into the van, I just flung the bag with the shirt over the two bench seats behind me. I gripped the wheel and let out the most primal scream I've ever uttered outside a birthing room. I remember looking up at the sky calling God a nasty piece of work (among other things that aren't fit to print) and I begged for the occurrences to stop long enough for me to catch my breath. I promised to take some time, really, really soon to figure out what I'm not facing that was causing this cascade of events.

I drove, shakily, back to the clinic and started to list the remedies in my head that I would do shooters of once I got back home. Mostly because I thought the quarter inch of vodka in the stock bottles might help too! *Aconite, Ignatia, NSOL, Lac Humanum*, and *Pulsatilla* were the few my misfiring brain could barely fathom.

As I dragged myself up the front steps, the European contingent were just departing. I wondered if they could detect that a mad woman was indeed running the Hahnemann College. I bid them good-bye and proceeded to cloister myself in my office to answer the phone calls and e-mails that had accumulated.

One e-mail was from a student who I'd grown quite close to asking for advice about her son who was still in terrible angst over his father's suicide. Her practitioner thought I might be able to help and she was guided to me. She illustrated some behavioural issues that she believed were manifesting due to his unresolved angst. I wrote her back and let her know that I could empathize and that I was still working on remnants of anger and grief from my mother's suicide from 30 years prior.

Each layer of this unfolding onion never ceases to amaze me and I was finally getting to a place that felt like just the other side of *Natrum Muriaticum* disease and even remotely resembled a celebration. The healthier I became, the thinner the barrier between this earth plane and the seeming other side. Every day, I was learning to reconnect with my mother through engaging with my abandoned sense of self. I told the student that I wasn't able to give this the thought and consideration that it deserved here at the office, but that I was forwarding it to my home where I would respond in a day or two.

I managed to take the Wednesday off before my sister-in-law arrived and the glorious bubbles in my steaming bath dampened the pages of my dirty little novel. I spent the day doing nothing other than what my spirit moved me to do. I took a long nap in the afternoon and even watched Oprah Winfrey at 4:00 p.m. before the kids tumbled through the door with the news of their day.

I came to realize what I was navigating during *Psorinum* 50M. It was the "tension" phase as in Wilhelm Reich's four-beat cycle. Now I don't know a whole lot about this from an intellectual perspective, but I kind of picked up the terms and meanings as my journey so nicely illustrated the subsequent charge, discharge and relaxation over the past year. The tension, to me, was the setting of the stage. During this phase of *Psora* I had to get so spent and worn down to become aware of my inability to surrender to my own inner truth. I have spent most of my life dancing in avoidance as I run around like an unglued chicken with all the doing in an effort to fulfill everyone's needs. I believed that if I was able to satiate all the noise first, that I could eventually get to my own needs which have been safely stored way up on a shelf in the back of my closet. This was an illusion, as the time never presented itself. I always coloured it with more noise.

For me, the key has been coming into the fullness and truer responsibility of self. *The Pulsatilla/Cancer* state of mind that led me to rescue everyone else to the exclusion of self suddenly became tiresome. I began to cut the cords of co-dependency in every unhealthy relationship I had fostered in my life. I learned to say "no" more emphatically until I was sure I was heard. As I did this I felt myself reel back into my own earthly shoes, so to speak, and people I hadn't talked to in years began calling me out of the blue to get together. It seemed they could sense on some level what I had done and they were looking to plug the needy chord back into my belly. No wonder I was so hungry that infamous day, my own spirit was starving! I continued to let them go and even had to go as far as to be very honest with a few of them as annoyance began bordering on harassment. I even changed my home phone number and to this day, I rarely feel a desire to interrupt my life to answer the phone.

This facet of my journey has been no walk in the park! I just about yearned myself out of existence during *Tuberculinum*, stopped sleeping from 3-5 a.m. during *Medhorrinum* (a sleepless mad woman who drove like a maniac), and landed very solidly into a grounded self during *Cancer* which I blew through in 48 hours. When I wrote this, I had only taken *Syphilinum* CM three days before, so I had yet to comment.

Over that past year, I had separated from my first husband, moved my son to a Waldorf school from a very sick public system (where we went down kicking and screaming all the way), and joyously been connected with my soul's mate. My newer theme was more about trust and surrender to the truth. In the past, I had conducted myself through the will to survive and it was time to let go a little more. I loved my new solo sneakers. They were white with gold and phosphorous glitter all over and bright purple laces. They have taken me from the realm of "lack" so characterized by *Psorinum* all the way to a truer realm of authenticity. And if you look carefully at the soles, you may see that they are pretty muddy! We've been through a lot!

CHAPTER 20

THE MERCURY AND YEAST CONNECTION

B y the third round of miasms, I only had one unresolved symptom left. I still suffered with chronic bladder and yeast infections. I knew that my faith in the medicine was sound as I was studying the principles and the medicine always affected cure. So why hadn't we been able to annihilate the root cause of this issue. Every month, I would welcome my period as this seemed to produce an alkaline state like a balm to the acid that tore my sensitive skin to ribbons over the course of the rest of the month.

I had used a *Candida Albicans* dropper for years with no change, in addition to going on a strict candida diet. My bladder and urethra burned as if my urine was as corrosive as battery acid. I had ingested every "*simillimum*", in every potency imaginable. Nothing seemed to touch it.

I went on my own personal research campaign which began with live blood analysis. In my opinion, this is one of the best diagnostic tools available to us. We can view our own inner cosmos on screen from one drop of blood that tells a detailed story from how much water and minerals we are absorbing to how much emotional and physical stress we're under. The results are undeniable and you can track your progress with treatment to gauge more visually how you are doing.

The Hahnemann College Clinic boasts one of the best live blood analysis clinics in the world. Linda Clifford can tell the most awesome details about your well-being from one drop of your blood on a slide under the "dark field" microscope. This is another way of viewing the blood which enables a practitioner to work more in the area of prevention. The light refraction allows you to view the active community of cells illustrating the biochemical and physiologic functions of your living internal milieu.

Alternatively, venous blood or "dead blood" cell analysis sent off to the lab by your allopathic doctor will measure red and white blood cell counts more effectively than dark field analysis. Immune deficiency, iron levels and hemoglobin tell more after you have unfortunately incurred disease.

Because we are animated beings, we house a living essence or spirit that is not measured as well by allopathic medicine. This is the aspect of self that is retained year after year even though every cell in our body effectively dies and is replaced by new ones. The animated principle is the part of us that remembers we had pink icing and rainbow sprinkles on our birthday cake a year ago! It is also the part of us that energetically cannot be created or destroyed, under any circumstances, even after the body's demise.

So there I was looking at a screen watching my beautiful red blood cells floating around freely and unencumbered. Linda pointed out the few clusters of yeast I had seen previously and I asked her what else she saw. She guided my attention to some heavy metal toxicity and suggested that I might do a heavy metal detox to see if that helped my specific condition. She also suggested that if I'd had mercury fillings, I might have retained mercury when they were filled.

I told her my mouth had been full of them, but that I had had them completely replaced about a year after Jordan was born. I now had gorgeous white amalgams which I explained to Linda would serve me well if I'd chosen to be an operatic Diva! I was disappointed to find out that my white amalgams carry their own toxic baggage.

Linda probed further and asked me if my dentist had properly "irrigated" my mouth with air to suck out the toxic fumes from the mercury extractions. I didn't know. Certainly my mouth had been "dammed" when they were extracted with a rubber-like trampoline that had made me gag, but I was unsure about the irrigation part.

Either way the timing made sense when I thought about it. I had chronic bladder and yeast infections in my teens about three to five years after having my entire mouth filled with mercury fillings and again more recently after having them all replaced. Could there be a link?

Linda suggested I do a heavy metal detoxification using the homeopathic remedies in addition to proper organ support. She cautioned me that this can be uncomfortable during the dumping stages and it is best done in the spring and fall months when you are consuming more seasonal vegetables which help in the detoxification process. I began taking chlorophyll, chlorella and cilantro drops which would effectively bind the yeast which encased the metals to encourage the dumping of the toxic elements out through my bowel as opposed to the kidneys. Mercury is particularly hard on the kidneys and could explain the corrosiveness I suffered monthly in my urogenital system. Also, the immune system will attack the kidneys during the detoxification process in an attempt to fight the inimical metals which can compromise the body's optimum immune functioning.

I began the regime, stuck to raw whole foods and doubled my water intake to effectively flush out my system. Even though I took only a 30CH containing the seven most common metals, by the second night I felt like a toxic waste dump. I had a headache, nausea, and my rib cage had swelled noticeably from my expanding liver as it worked to dump the toxins

I paced the floor through some of the night, holding myself like I was rocking a newborn. The taste of metal leeched into my mouth through my saliva. I thought a lot about my long plight with mercury and the anger surfaced which provoked me to write the following poem in June, 2003:

Mecurius

The terror pricks up my spine as I face the beige leather chair,
the trays glistening with metallic instruments, medieval torture

The light glares down and my eyes tear feathers from the corners
his breath presses through the thick entanglement of reddish nose hair

Glimpses of his thick salivating tongue, the fetid breath reaches for me
and the needle is drawn from behind his back, my scream in abeyance

My eyes squeeze shut, my jaw is pried open and the pricks render the
chemical rage that will numb my rose coloured estuary, I moan with fear

Bristling hairy hands deliver the mercury divorced of its natal ore
and the slimy dissolving solvent of Quicksilver fuses to my enamelled spirit

The day before, I had run like The Mariner, a winged messenger through the grass
with Apollo and Hermes in the glinting sun en route to the evening star

Today I am subject to the God of Commerce and thievery as my thirteen year
old molars receive the mawkish liquescent toxicity that will define my bane

For twenty-seven years hence I've suffered with acute inflammation of the brain,
acridity from every orifice and voluptuous itching that characterized my intimacy.

Great were the demands for sugar to feed the yeast which housed the mercury
to prevent the ultimate poisoning whose toxicity had obviously killed the rat

"and this is the woman all tattered and torn
who lays in the house that Jack built"

Clarke's Materia Medica cites "Fits of mania and dementia with a disposition to
anger, weakness of memory, loss of willpower and flights into rage and passion"

I have also known the screaming urethra, the copious corrosive urine,
and raw and excoriated labia with Mammae so sore and swollen
they prepare to ulcerate into full bloom Peonies

As I cleanse the lethal poison from my body, my overburdened liver
threatens to squeeze out between my ribs, my abdomen tears at my back
and my armpits bulge their hinges

The murderous panic consumes my restless anguish and all at once,
I am driven to walk for miles in search of my tormentor,
the allopathic King pin of the one with the hairy nose and the fetid breath

On this day, the suspicious quarrelsome humour drops onto the page and the
mercurial tears wash away the semblance of disease incurred over lifetimes, the
mucus scalds my nose for the last time

Last time you peeked through the curtains of my bedchamber
with the tiny bottle held fast beneath your cloak,
the unraveling truths raised now for my conscious understanding

Our rotational orbits will not cross in resonance again;
your theory of relativity is now traveling at a slightly different pace than mine.

After a couple of weeks, I felt I was on the other side of this healing reaction. My mental acuity increased tenfold due to the fact that mercury and the yeast that encases it, sits in the cavity of the brain. My bladder and yeast infections have only appeared once in almost a year when I went up in the next potency.

Essentially, the yeast is just an indicator of the presence of heavy metals in the body's milieu. The craving for sugar is a call to feed the yeast which might explain why so many individuals who suffer fungi infections also crave carbohydrates.

In essence, when the allopathic community sends in anti-fungal antibiotics like Nystatin™, a sulpha-based drug, it suppresses the yeast effectively driving the root cause into the body one more layer. Essentially, the wrong enemy is being confronted and this is why patients and their doctors admit that yeast is one of the most difficult to address. Homeopathy gets to the root of the problem.

CHAPTER 21

BREAST TUMOUR?

In January of 2003, I was out in Victoria, British Columbia working for the Hahnemann College at The Victoria Health Show. I was staying with a friend in her beautiful home nestled amongst the trees on the side of a mountain where we hiked daily. She said it was a "hill" by Western standards, but I still called it a "mountain" every time I hiked straight up the side of it!

The difference in the time zones caused me to waken at five o'clock every morning and I would use the time to study the Regimen Module of my course. Two days earlier, on the plane coming west, I had read about Heilkunst treatment of tumours and cancer.

It was on one of these early mornings that I lay in bed thinking about the fruit salad I was going to have for breakfast when I noticed a sensation in my left breast. It was a dull ache. My period had just ended so this feeling did not coincide with the usual post-menstrual sensations.

I placed my hand on my breast and was immediately drawn to a tender orb about one inch in circumference. I checked the right breast to see if I was mistaken. The mottled surface resembling the moon was quite normal on the right and the left did indeed contain an obvious lump. As the realization of the tumour surfaced in waves, I began to ponder what unconscious message it was here to purvey. Through my Heilkunst treatment, I had learned to try to scope out the meaning of illness before rattling my "therapeutic cage."

I got up before anyone else woke and I began to walk the mountain taking the long route. I descended into the dark tropical forest that was dank and musky with moss and ferns covering every surface between Douglas firs so massive my Sport Utility would have been eclipsed.

As I walked the forest floor, I felt the hot tears rising up into my throat. Could it be I had been forsaken by the medicine? Had I come all this way to also be forsaken by God and plucked from the earth plane just as I was finding my authentic self? What about the book I was writing about the medicine? Wasn't this about me realizing my life's purpose to bridge the medicine to others out of the hands of academia? Were my children also destined to live a motherless existence? Was my separation from their father a year ago now going to push their trauma quotient over the top?

No answers were spoken by the mountain, and so I let the tears fill in the spaces between the questions and I continued to walk. By this time, the sun began to poke beams of light through dense foliage to form a crystalline splendour on leaves holding plump droplets of dew. If I were a woodland fairy, I would have found my eternal home there.

The path began to ascend and I hiked straight up for a mile or two until the trees began to thin and the sun warmed my face fully. I looked across the salty strait to snow-capped mountains of the United States. Bands of morning clouds not yet burnt off by the sun, hung like shades while the peaks finished dressing for the day.

I was feeling better as I welcomed the warmth on my skin while still feeling the cool shadows clinging to my hiking boots from below. Further above the tree line, I climbed, lungs panting with the bodily effort and my spirit quieted with the reassurance of nature's abundance. As I reached the pinnacle, I turned in a circle to view Mt. Baker and Mt. St. Helen's. This was not the first or last time I would be challenged. I knew that the tumour had a story to tell and I would just have to sit myself down and listen carefully. As I stood at the top overlooking the view, a glorious Monarch sailed by. The red/orange of her wings against the baby blue sky was breathtaking.

Two days later, I flew home to Ottawa to continue ruminating on the action to take. Two weeks later, I told my partner Jeff what I discovered. He was so calm and centered that I felt reassured by his reaction. He accompanied me back to Linda Clifford and Live Blood Analysis. Indeed, the tumour registered on screen. The telltale signs of the presence of cancer were in my cells, and indicated a higher level of sodium than potassium and that my alkalinity was too low and being replaced by acid. Linda calmly took my hands and told me what my options were in addition to using homeopathic remedies.

I knew from my studies that a number of individuals had been working at curing cancer for years. Roy Rife used the frequency instrument treatment by aligning short waves of light and longer waves of light into a tube which is the energetic simillimum of the virus or bacteria.

Dr. Gerson[27] understood that microbes in cancer patients changed and he wrote that it is a "biological fact that not one factor alone or a combination of single factors is decisive but what is decisive is how they influence the whole body, mind and soul in their entirety." Again, he sees the common element of the nature of disease and that is what he goes after with his juicing of organic fruits and vegetables, and coffee enemas.

Dr. Enderlein[28] proved using a dark-field microscope that micro-organisms in the human body can develop from apathogenic forms to pathogenic forms due exclusively to the patient's "milieu interieur" (internal environment). He noted that the acid/alkaline balance was determined by the organism's protein content – an imbalance in the Astral and Etheric bodies (Light and Dark).

Dr. Naessens[29] observed that the cancer cell was ultimately a process of primitive fermentation (anabolic respiration). By observing the cycle of a somatid (concentration of energy) where, through process, normal genetic properties are transmissible to living organisms which materialize in the Leib. He further noted that in absence of this three-phase cycle, no cellular division can occur. If what I understood was correct, Dr. Naessens introduced healthy somatids to his patients (Formula 714X) which stimulated the immune response by reversing the sclerotic or dying tendency of the lymphatic system.

Dr. Chachoua[30] discovered that if he created a "nemesis" agent like cold, flu or even cells containing syphilis, he could "tag" these less invasive cells onto the cancer cells of a patient. Since the immune system doesn't recognize or adequately deal with cancer cells, Dr. Chachoua attached natural disease agents that are inimical to the cancer virus.

I booked an appointment with Rudi Verspoor as I wanted the "ringmaster" of Heilkunst operations! I was scared and I needed him to explain to me how I had grown a breast tumour in the face of my treatment. Surely, it would not bear well for business if the registrar of your Homeopathic College should bite the dust from cancer.

I tearfully explained my condition and Rudi engaged me gently and spoke calmly in a quiet reassuring tone. He said, "Ally, your body is just following the direction of cure!" I looked at him like he had horns on his head, and I fired back an indignant, "What?!" He repeated, "Your body is just following the direction of cure. You've left a stagnating marriage and are taking full possession of self and the tumour is just doing its job by mopping up the spiritual and emotional toxicity of the past 12 years. You spent all that time trying to rescue your husband, his family and even your children and you have now effectively let go!" He continued by saying, "Now that you are fully embodying your life's path and fully assuming responsibility for self, it is natural for your body to develop a physical manifestation of the work you've done towards cure."

I sat back, relaxed a little and cocked my head to eye him skeptically. "You mean to tell me that the tumour is just an indication that my body is healing itself?" Rudi nodded and continued, by telling me that cancer is just another inflammatory response that gets caught replicating cells on its way to our consciousness. If the energy gets blocked repeatedly due to avoidance tactics, the energy starts to replicate on the cellular level at an alarming rate. Rather than choosing to carve our tumours out of our bodies, we can learn their meaning for us, treat the underlying cause, gain the consciousness and effectively move forward with our lives.

So, I asked Rudi how much regimen I should employ. Should I juice 25 lb. bags of carrots until my skin turned orange and my cells were convinced otherwise? He said either way, my body would cure itself now that I had the realization and the tumour would just continue to follow the direction of cure out to the surface and beyond. I wanted to believe him, but I was still cautious so I asked him if I should use the homeopathic remedies at a minimum. Again, he reiterated that the tumour would go away on its own and that I could employ any therapeutic tactic I wanted in the interim.

I admit that my organs of trust were not as profoundly honed as Rudi's. I went out and bought the cadillac of juicers and Jeff lovingly made carrot juice for me twice a day. I wanted to approach this situation like a scientist so every night we measured the tumour with our fingers and recorded the data.

I interviewed all eight Heilkunst doctors to find out their success with cancer. I learned that in all cases, tumours were indeed just disappearing. In one case, the tumour moved from the patient's left breast to the centre of her chest, a small opening appeared in the skin and the tumour actually emerged out through the opening in the skin. I was flabbergasted.

I completely surrounded myself with calm reassuring friends and colleagues delighting in their stories about cure. Many of them called me every day to find out how I was doing. Throughout those weeks, I only had doubt planted in my mind once by a family member who thought I should have a biopsy.

On that evening, I began to take the homoeopathic remedies *Conium, Carbo Animalis* and *Phytolacca.* Jeff and I both noticed that the tumour had increased in mass. Two nights later, it had doubled in size and was in fact losing its hardened defined shape.

By the third night, I could feel a strand had spawned off the tumour down towards my organs. I juiced, ate only whole raw foods, and took the remedies to encourage lymphatic drainage. The toxins were moving and I was feeling quite tired. I felt invited to nap in the afternoon and sleep at least ten hours every night.

By the fifth day, although my breast was still tender, we could not detect the tumour at all. At six weeks from the day I had first detected the lump, the entire issue had effectively been annihilated by my very amazing body. No sensation remained at all. Oh, how I celebrated the renewal of my glorious life!

I learned more about love, support and trust of self during that voyage with my tumour. I had effectively surrounded myself with the mirror images of what I felt I deserved. I learned again to step one more step away from allopathic thinking to embrace every iota of my being even if it begins with 'C'. I had learned to fall in love with the wisdom carried by my tumour and trust that she knew where she was going.

It was a part of me and represented the inflammatory response to years of trying to avoid becoming conscious. Heilkunst prevailed; my faith was once again restored. I realized again that it is so much more about the purveyors of this system of medicine and less about the remedies themselves. You have to be healthy enough to sustain the charge that fear brings from the shadow of our beings.

Would I ever be competent and healthy enough to look into the face of a cancer patient and calmly and compassionately point out the direction for cure? Certainly, it was something I could shoot for on the other side of the moon!

CHAPTER 22

FACING THE SHADOW

In the Hebrew Scriptures, Isaiah says: "Woe unto them that call evil good, and good evil; that put darkness for light, and light for darkness; that put bitter for sweet, and sweet for bitter ... Therefore is the anger of the Lord kindled against his people."

The twin forces of good and evil, light and dark, appear in most traditions with variations on the theme. In Chinese Taoism, the well-known yin-yang symbol represents the alliance of opposites as they flow into one another; but in addition each pole contains the other in eternal embrace, inextricably linked by their very nature. Everything with substance casts a shadow.

I was learning that as I ascended out of the pain of physical symptoms my soul/spiritual journey was heading in an entirely different direction. Out of disease, I had sustained environmental stresses and pressures, which had helped me to create a great number of illusions and delusions to power my existence to date. Every issue I faced in an effort to becoming more conscious was like pulling another untruth from the magician's black bag of tricks. There wasn't a white rabbit to be found!

I faced the fact that I had attempted to mother my younger sister after our mother's death in an effort to mother myself. I did a very poor job of both and she was naturally resentful of my self-appointment. I found that I had to destroy the illusion, sustain the demotion and just go about being her sister again to properly honour our relationship. I reveled in the new "lack" of responsibility and I saw that she was more than capable of taking care of herself.

We all have a shadow. Or does the shadow have us? Carl Jung turned this question into a riddle when he asked: "How do you find a lion that has swallowed you?" In essence, I was realizing as I was uncomfortably knocking around in the dark, and although I could feel his ribs, I had no clue where I was with respect to my healing. No map or light to read it by!

I began reading anything written by Rudolf Steiner.[31] I was introduced to *How to Know Higher Worlds* through a group interested in discovering Anthroposophy and I began to chart a course for myself. It was critical to me that by going through the process of destroying states of mind born out of disease that I not just replace one false belief with another. Steiner does an awesome job of providing the framework for moving through the Shadowlands. The details, the colours and the way were naturally born out of my inner process. While some may need to invoke their will to move forward, it was intrinsic for me to find a way to surrender. What if there was no net? Some days, I flip-flopped hourly between faith and fear.

Through this process, I was running headlong into unrecognized desires and repressed portions of my personality. In the psychological atmosphere created by parents, siblings, caretakers, and other important sources of love and approval, I was supposed to have begun the necessary process of ego development long before now. Human adaptation to society and the world requires the creation of an ego, an "I", to serve as the organizing principle of a growing consciousness. I had no idea who that "I" was and my health and well-being demanded I find out. Now was the time and my false ego had to go!

Ego development depends upon our repressing what is "wrong" or "bad" in us, while we identify with what is perceived and reinforced as good. This positive incarnation of the "I" can provide the growing personality a strategic advantage in eliminating anxiety and winning positive regard. The process of growing a healthy ego continues throughout the first half of life, modified by external influences and experiences as we move out into the world.

As ego comes, so goes the shadow: the disowned self is a natural by-product of the ego-building process, and the two of us weren't going to be passing each other like two innocent ships in the night. There were many icebergs and I was having some pretty phenomenal dreams, visions and images as I grappled with the dark side that was emerging from within. Also the physical sensations were interesting.

The first night that I went into *Stramonium*, I was staying at Jeff's apartment. It was a hot night in July and the fan was on full blast in an attempt to stay cool. The lights in the courtyard outside the window were on motion detectors and suddenly switched off. It was about 4:00 a.m. In the darkness black as pitch, I turned around and imagined that the pin in the fan blade had just popped out. The metal blade released from the casing and was hurling across the room to carve me up into small morsels. The terror was primal and I screamed as the fear enveloped me. Jeff flipped on the light and the fan was naturally still wholly intact. I took the remedy *Stramonium* and went back to sleep. I have never forgotten how I felt in that moment and was able to spot the state clearly in a patient of my own very recently.

Unbeknownst to me at the time I entered treatment, there are two other realms defined by Heilkunst: the Chthonic Realm, of which *Stramonium* is one of the states, and the *Ideogenic*. The first is really where your fears reside which I've illustrated as the shadow. Fears are really a function of our ignorance. For example, I took on the role of my sister's mother in an attempt to fill in my own gap where further nurturing would not be forthcoming. I assumed that she would naturally crave this and by acting as her self-appointed guardian, I was attempting to stave off the fear that had become intrinsic to my existence. Eventually this core belief caught up to me and I was dethroned. I remember how shocked I was at the realization that I had attempted to address my own void by attempting to fill another's.

I also have always had a strong feeling of self-righteousness which is also an over-compensation for the fear I have of "not being enough." This stemmed from my mother's suicide and I always believed if I had told her I loved her that morning, before she died, she might have stayed with me.

Waltzing in these new realms is a little like when Hahnemann couldn't figure out why his patients weren't being cured long term before he unearthed the chronic miasms. The *Chthonic* realm was identified by Rudi Verspoor and Steven Decker out of clinical research done by Paul Herscu[32] and subsequently more extensive observations by Rudi Verspoor, since many patients were encountering their fears as they stripped away their timeline events and subsequently their genetic miasms.

The *Ideogenic* realm is the realm of spiritual diseases and the current final frontier so to speak. In my limited experience, they often are illumined after a dance or two through the *Chthonic* Realm. Again, research is limited, but I have had an affectionate waltz in both these arenas and can attest that I have counted the ribs of my lion a few times now. The interesting fact about the *Ideogenic* realm is that if the beliefs are fairly new and not too entrenched, they can be annihilated using the law of opposites. By offering a piece of verbal "truth," it can counteract the disease and annihilate it.

I never thought of myself as a fearful person. In fact, I admired my own strength and courage to overcome obstacles and exact my will at times when required. My personal mantra has been "Courage To Be" since my headmaster illuminated this message from classical literature in high school. So, I was the most surprised to find that I had been operating out of fear and ignorance as a product of my disease states for most of my life. The interesting challenge is how these primal fears are being played out in all our lives by our brethren. From those individuals living in the streets up to the corporate executive, the media exploits our fears dampening our collective "Courage To Be."

It made sense to me to be facing these issues in a safe, supportive environment where I felt free to express them unbridled. It was paramount to me that these doctors of homeopathic medicine had done the same in their own paths to cure too. Only through true empathy did I find my path and thankfully Patty and Rudi had gone before us to pave the way!

The darkness contains the etheric forces that power the growth of plants. Think of the seed of a sunflower in spring as you bury it in the earth. By August, the plant can be over six feet tall with a stalk as thick as your thumb. Astrality, or your desires, is derived from the cosmos. Animals are an illustration of astral beings. Instincts derived by the lion will drive her to hunt for food, mate and care for her young. The ego is also a function of the cosmos and the physical body is your vehicle of dense matter residing on the earth.

True remediation and health is really about descending through the four bodies in the order of Ego, Astral, Etheric and Physical while resolving any overdue accounts with the Universe. Steven Decker defines it as the Descent of Gnosis (Spirit). Only then can an individual ascend into a state of newer consciousness where the star ship Enterprise has never been before! The tightrope across the chasm between light and dark can be filled with sceptres from the *Chthonic* and *Ideogenic* realms. But when the ascension finally occurs up into a new state of consciousness through the newly defined Physical, Etheric, Astral and into the true sense of "I," the sense of humility and omnipotence is more profound than ever imagined. This is a new state of consciousness traversed by few and those that have arrived there won't be found on street corners touting messages from the anti-Christ. This is a profoundly solo journey and there are very few versed guides to this uncharted Garden of Eden. True ascension demands nothing less as the lion must be slayed one rib at a time from the inside out.

CHAPTER 23

WHERE TO GO FROM HERE?

Paracelsus, the 16th-century Swiss alchemist-physician, wrote: "God has not permitted any disease without providing a remedy. Only ignoramuses allege that Nature has not provided a remedy against every disease."[33] This maxim is bizarrely confirmed in the widely held suspicion that Acquired Immune Deficiency Syndrome, AIDS, may have been developed in a government laboratory for the purposes of selective population control; a modern abomination remnant of Hitler's regime.

Richard Leviton cites that allopathy faces a conceptual dead end called AIDS as there is no capacity in its midst to cure this disease. Essentially, you can't transplant an autoimmune system, and chemotherapeutics and antibiotics will only hasten the demise of these patients as their immune systems are further compromised. We don't have to be terribly conscious to realize the word "anti" means against and "bios" is life.

Leviton illustrates the allopathic thinking, "Now, if you transfuse billions of healthy bone-marrow-generated white blood cells (containing killer T-cells, trained to respond to cytomegalovirus) into a leukemia, cancer or

AIDS patient, allopathic logic itself argues that you'll need to inject anti-rejection, immune-suppressant drugs at the same time, to prevent the recipient's immune system from rejecting the foreign T-cells."[34]

In essence what he is saying is that for allopathy to work, you have to suppress the recipient's immune response so his or her immune system can receive an immune enhancer. No gain is possible, as the double negative collapses under scrutiny; the medical logic undermines the therapeutic value, which just ends in a heap of contradictions and the patient's demise.

"Allopathy will end up destroying the immune system even faster than AIDS," says Leviton, "and this is because we are dealing with the nature of immunology, and it is time we admit that we have reached the threshold of the mystery of being human."[35] We are dynamic, interactive, animated spirit beings that possess identities greater than competent killer T-cells.

Dr. Deepak Chopra also supports that you can't transplant a person. You don't need $10 billion to figure that out. "It's no different than the final surprise awaiting particle physicists and their multibillion-dollar supercolliders: the ultimate particle is consciousness itself."[36] Chopra says that "physicists will discover this the minute they accept their role in the making of the particles they are observing. The Physicist makes particles that physical reality participates in the mind of the physicist. Someday, we may realize that we have been looking in a mirror all along!"[37]

A woman in the United States was diagnosed with AIDS. She leaves her stagnant job to live out her last apportioned six months doing precisely what she feels she was always destined to do. She begins to paint murals. She travels around the country making bold statements of colour and conception on walls and billboards of towns and cities. Nine months tick by, and then a year and she can't figure out what happened to her death sentence. She checks into a local clinic for a blood work-up and her AIDS is entirely gone. Effectively, the shadow has been replaced by the healthy ego. We've heard about these non-researched cases with countless diseases including Cancer and now AIDS. Spontaneous remission is not an illusion; it is a function of increased consciousness.

Leviton goes on to cite that, "The cure for AIDS is, literally, a new person, re-created through Consciousness."[38]   The effective downloading of Ego! In essence, allopathy is the intellectual vacuum that deadens the "I" and when we start to wake up to this truth, we will realize we are truly embroiled in the unsuspected battle for human freedom. "Allopathy may have generated the very wedge that cracks open its own deadly and deadening edifice.   If AIDS is human made, this raises the stakes in the immunological struggle to incarnate an authentic human identity (Steiner's Ego) in the human organism, but it doesn't change the basic issue."[39]

Our battle for freedom is illustrated in our efforts to spiritualize our material life. We have the right to become conscious. Beginning in 1945, the U.S. Army's Project Paperclip recruited, protected and financed more that 2,000 Nazi war criminals and "mad scientists" for work in the U.S. defence and intelligence industries. Dr. Leonard Horowitz's research in his book *Emerging Viruses, AIDS and Ebola – Nature, Accident or Genocide?* unveiled a secret agreement among NATO, NASA, and a Nazi-linked West German company called OTRAG to lease 29,000 square miles of eastern Zaire (inhabited by 760,000 people) for military purposes. "This area is very close to what is now known as "The AIDS Highway" and the eruption point for Ebola virus. The Zairian site might have been ground zero for both diseases," says Dr. Horowitz."[40]

In the 1970s the toxic AIDS virus may have been inserted into hepatitis B and smallpox vaccine trials in Zaire (in children), New York City (1,083 gay men) and San Francisco (7,000 gay men). Dr. Horowitz says that the U.S. government is to blame and must take responsibility for these experimental and production vaccines being contaminated by the deadly toxins, giving rise to mutated virus strains. It is time this biological Trojan horse be raised up for our viewing consciousness and then gutted and dismantled.

On a much smaller scale, but no less important, a man arrived in my clinic very recently and said that he was scared to enter the local allopathic medical clinic in his neighbourhood. Apparently, the last time he was there, he waited over 45 minutes; the doctor saw him for a total of two minutes and provided him with a prescription for high blood pressure.

When my patient checked the interrelationship with the new drug against the one he was currently on, using the Internet, there was a significant contra-indication that could provoke a heart attack. This patient was a healthy young male and former athlete and he expressed a great deal of grief and anger over having lost his stamina to the current drug therapy and said, "First they take away my freedom, and now they threaten my life too. This can't be the right way to treat people."

Incidentally, this patient had never heard of homeopathy until recently and was recommended to me by a friend. After I explained the principles and philosophy of treatment, he told me that although he was skeptical, it seemed to make sense. I look forward to the day that his cholesterol is reduced and he is off all medication and his freedom is also restored to a state of cure.

I sometimes wonder how a middle-aged woman in suburbia, Ottawa, who survived the premature birth of her son, a case of PMS, and a breast tumour became so fascinated with medicine and the battle for human freedom. I guess it was while I was connecting the ribs of my own lion, I noticed a broader context for humanity. I am so thankful for the gift of discernment, which was born out of restoring my health. As a result, I have been able to tap into a global community of authentic truth seekers who have also connected these same dots, driving their consciousness forward. These illuminated souls walk so tall before me to the land of freedom. This is *The Path To Cure, The Whole Art of Healing* as I have grown to know it. My love and thanks be to God and to Jordan Ephraim, born July 23, 1993 on the day of the double rainbow, who helped me to begin my descent down and then up this path of true enlightenment in order to find my true "Courage To Be."

If only it were all so simple! If only there were evil people somewhere insidiously committing evil deeds, and it were necessary only to separate them from the rest of us and destroy them. But the line dividing good and evil cuts through the heart of every human being.
And who is willing to destroy a piece of his own heart?

Alexander Solzhenitsyn

ENDNOTES

1. Brennan, Barbara Ann, *Light Emerging, The Journey of Personal Healing*, Bantam, 1988.

2. Verspoor, Rudolf, HD(RHom), Decker, Steven, *The Dynamic Legacy: From Homeopathy to Heilkunst, An ongoing Study of the Meaning in the Writings of Samuel Hahnemann within the Context of the Dynamic System of Thought, Leading Thereby to a More Powerful System of Cure for Disease*, Hahnemann College for Heilkunst Press, 2000.

3. Hahnemann, Samuel, MD, edited and annotated by Wenda Brewster O'Reilly, PhD, *Organon of the Medical Art*, Birdcage Books, 1996, p.25.

4. Elmiger, Jean, MD, *Rediscovering Real Medicine, The New Horizons of Homeopathy*, Elements Books, Great Britain, Text, 1998.

5. Hahnemann, Samuel, MD, ibid, p. 65.

6. Gibson, Douglas, MD, Edited by Marianne Harling, MD, Brian Kaplan, MD, *Studies of Homeopathic Remedies*, The Homeopathic Trust, London, 1987.

7. Hahnemann, Samuel, MD, ibid, p. 60.

8. Verspoor, Rudolf, HD(RHom), Decker, Steven, 2000, ibid, electronic library.

9. Verspoor, Rudolf, HD(RHom), Decker, Steven, 2000, ibid, electronic library.

10. Verspoor, Rudolf, HD(RHom), Decker, Steven, 2000, ibid, electronic library.

11. Verspoor, Rudolf, HD(RHom), Decker, Steven, 2000, ibid, electronic library.

12. Gibson, Douglas, 1987, ibid, p. 469.

13. Goleman, Daniel, PhD, *Emotional Intelligence: Why It Can Matter More Than IQ for Character, Health and Lifelong Achievement*, www.eiconsortium.org/members/goleman.htm, June 2, 1997.

14. Gibson, Douglas, 1987, ibid, p. 413.

15. Gibson, Douglas, 1987, ibid, p. 110.

16. Verspoor, Rudolf, HD(RHom), 2000, ibid, electronic library.

17. Chia, Mantak, Abrams, Douglas, *The multi-Orgasmic Man*, Harper Collins, San Francisco, 1997.

18. Chia, Mantak, Chia, Maneewan, *Healing Love Through the Tao, Cultivating Female Sexual Energy*, Healing Tao Books, 1986.

19. Morrison, Roger, MD, *Morrison's Desktop Guide to Keynotes and Confirmatory Symptoms*, Hahnemann Clinic Publishing, 1993.

20. Morrison, Roger, 1993, ibid, p. 376.

21. Nye, David, MD, Quote derived from Fibromyalgia Support Site, http//fibromyalgia.ncf.ca/

22. Dethlefsen, Thorwald, *The Healing Power of Illness*, English Translation by Peter Lemesturier, Element Books Limited, 1990.

23. Singh, Narayan, *Messages From The Body*, N. Singh Publishing, 1997.

24. Smith, Patty, HD(RHom),Verspoor, Rudolf, HD(RHom.), *The Heilkunst Journal*, The Hahnemann College for Heilkunst, illustrating continuing research and personal stories of patients, 1996 – ongoing.

25. Verspoor, Rudolf, HD(RHom)

26. Singh, Narayan, ibid, Electronic Library.

27. Verspoor, Rudolf, HD(RHom), Gerson, Max, MD, 2000, ibid, Electronic Library.

28. Verspoor, Rudolf, HD(RHom), Enderlein, Günther MD, 2000, ibid, Electronic Library.

29. Verspoor, Rudolf, HD(RHom), Naessens, Gaston, MD, 2000, ibid, Electronic Library.

30. Verspoor, Rudolf, HD(RHom), Chachoua, Sam, MD, 2000, ibid, Electronic Library.

31. Steiner, Rudolf (1861-1925) Austrian born scientific, literary and philosophical scholar, particularly known for his work on Goethe's scientific writings.

32. Paul Herscu, ND, a native of Romania, is a graduate of the National College of Naturopathic Medicine, in Portland, Orogon. He has written two books entitled *Stramonium and The Homeopathic Treatment of Children: Pediatric Constitutional Types.*

33. Leviton, Richard, prolific natural health Journalist since 1979, Richard Leviton is the author of six books, including *Looking for Arthur: A Once and Future Travelogue; The Imagination of Pentecost: Rudolf Steiner and Contemporary Spirituality,* and *Brain Builders! A Lifelong Guide to Sharper Thinking, Better Memory, and an Age-Proof Mind.* He lives, writes and edits in Virginia, p.153.

34. Leviton, Richard, ibid, p.142.

35. Leviton, Richard, *Physician, Medicine and the Unsuspected Battle for Human Freedon*, Hampton Roads Publishing Company Inc., 2000, p. 142.

36. Leviton, Richard, ibid, p. 143.

37. Leviton, Richard, ibid, p. 143.

38. Leviton, Richard, ibid, p. 147.

39. Leviton, Richard, ibid, p. 147.

40. Leviton, Richard, ibid, p. 154.

The
Path
to
Cure

The Whole Art of Healing

•

Allyson McQuinn devotes her life
to helping people heal.

•

To contact *Allyson McQuinn*
or order additional copies of this book,
please go to

www.arcanum.ca

•

Natural Medicine

598966095

About The Path to Cure

Many of us have experienced short-term m[...] the underlying cause flare up when least expe[...] e is indeed possible.

McQuinn takes readers on an intimate journey, showing how she came through homeopathic medicine to the broader system of Heilkunst (Healing Art) through her son's serious physical and behavioural problems. As her son improved dramatically and permanently, Allyson wondered what the medicine might hold to address her own issues. This book is a must-read if you want a life of health and wholeness for you and your loved ones.

About the Author

Allyson McQuinn, has been exploring homeopathy for almost ten years.

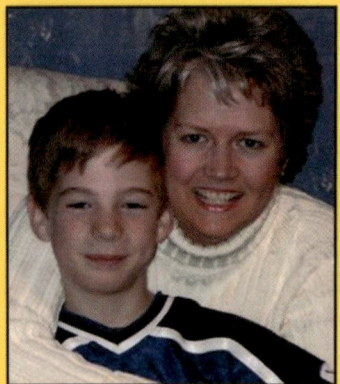

During her studies at the Hahnemann College for Heilkunst, McQuinn learned how to affect cure, why it works and how to repeat the results with all of her patients.

Allyson practises Heilkunst homeopathy in Ottawa, where she furthers her research in resonant partnership with her husband, Jeff Korentayer, also a doctor of homeopathic medicine. Her two healthy, awesome children, Jordan and Adie, are an infinite source of energy and wonder who remind her how important it is to take time out "to play." Allyson is currently writing two other books: a collection of her poetry and an approach to Heilkunst for children.

When we travel through an unknown country we trust our guide book. Allyson McQuinn has so gently and intimately written a guide book to take us through our inner country, the mysterious journey of health and healing.

Dr Farid Shodjaee, BSc, DDS

This book presents a comprehensive explanation of homeopathy. It is full of honesty, heartfelt emotion and provides a clear description of the healing process. I highly recommend it to anyone who wants to be truly well.

Mary Rothschild, MSW, RSW, DHHP, HD(RHom)

Providing you with powerful
information an[...]
book illustrates[...]
indeed possible[...]

ISBN 0-9735207-0-1

9780973520705

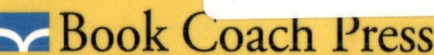

Book Coach Press

$24.00 CDN/$20.00 US